JERRY ANDERSON'S

# JOY OF FITNESS
## FOR WOMEN

## The Best and Easiest
## Way to Gain
## a Healthy Body
## and
## Peace of Mind

By Jerry L. Anderson
Mr. Natural Universe 1998

# Jerry Anderson's
# Joy of Fitness
# For Women

Copyright © Jerry Anderson 2000

Published by:  Apex Fitness House
4102 Orange Ave.
Suite 107-183
Long Beach, CA 90807

ISBN: 0-9677093-0-X

Library of Congress Card Catalog Number: 99-98089
Printed in the United States of America
10 9 8 7 6 5 4 3 2 1

Cover and Page design by One-On-One Book Production, West Hills, California

**PLEASE NOTE:** This book is not intended to take the place of medical advice and treatment from your personal physician. Readers are to consult their own doctor or other qualified professional regarding the treatment of their medical problems. Neither the publisher nor the author takes any responsibility for any possible consequences from any exercise or nutrition advice to any person reading or following the information in this book.

# CONTENTS

# CONTENTS (CONTINUED)

# ACKNOWLEDGMENTS

I WOULD LIKE TO THANK the following contributors for sharing their advice and insights:

God, for the wisdom and truth that lights my path.

Mom and Dad, for having me.

Shah, Andrew, Abdul, Jeff, William and Maxine for strong family support.

Family and friends, for encouragement, enthusiasm, and support.

Joe Weider, for providing so much fitness information in your highly successful *Muscle and Fitness* magazine and other fine publications.

Robin Sandoval, for the outstanding fitness modeling.

Stephanie Quenga, for the outstanding fitness modeling.

Martin Barajas, for the great photography.

David Lester, for your technical assistance.

Craig Givens, for computer expertise.

Marsha McClamb, for your wonderful insight and feedback from your Hair Plus Salon.

Star Baily D.C., contributing editor.

Kristina Coultrup, for the motivation and push.

Butch Dennis for his friendship and assistance.

Carolyn Porter and Alan Gadney for your book production expertise.

Otomix Footwear, for supplying the great looking workout shoes. For ordering information or a catalog, call 1-800-701-7867.

Hot Skins Bodywear, for supplying the great looking workout clothes. For ordering information or a catalog, call 1-800-775-2595.

Gay Givens, for being so motivating and supportive.

Ashley and Haley, for being so wonderful.

# ABOUT THE AUTHOR

* Mr. Natural Universe 1998
* Body-shaping Expert
* Fitness Expert
* Mr. Natural Southern California
* ACBA Head Judge
* Trainer of Champions
* ABA Athlete of the Year
* ABA Poser of the Year
* ACE Certified Personal Trainer
* AFFAA Certified Personal Trainer
* 16 Years Experience as Personal Trainer
* Television Commentator
* Motivation Expert
* Named by ACBA as "SUPER TRAINER"

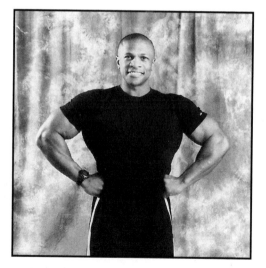

# INTRODUCTION

My goal in writing this book is to motivate women to eat healthy foods, exercise regularly and reduce unwanted body fat. My personal commitment is to help you embrace exercise and proper nutrition as a part of your lifestyle, thereby maintaining your natural health and beauty and improving your quality of life.

*Jerry Anderson's Joy of Fitness for Women* is written with sixteen years of successful body-shaping experience and nutritional success formulas. My programs will make exercise and healthy eating fun and pleasurable as you exercise your way to a healthy, fit and beautiful body.

Please write me when *Jerry Anderson's Joy of Fitness for Women* has improved your health and the quality of your life.

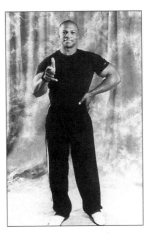

**Jerry L. Anderson**
**Mr. Natural Universe 1998**

My programs of exercise and nutrition are designed around scientific principles. The exercises used in this bodyshaping program are those that require the least amount of time and produce the greatest results.

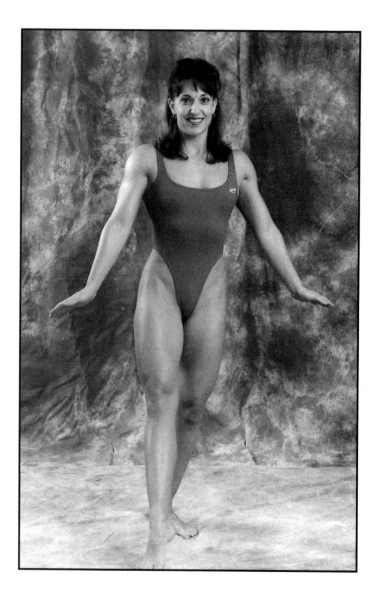

As you increase your strength on each exercise, you will automatically improve the shape, tone and definition of your muscles. Additionally, by following the nutrition success formula, you are guaranteed to reach your fat loss goals and become very happy and healthy in the process.

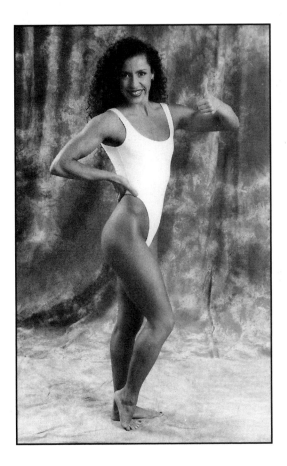

*       *       *

This program is ideal for women who want to reduce body fat, add shape and tone, and improve their health and fitness in the privacy of their own home, office or gym. For maximum results, I recommend using my program two to three times per week on non-consecutive days.

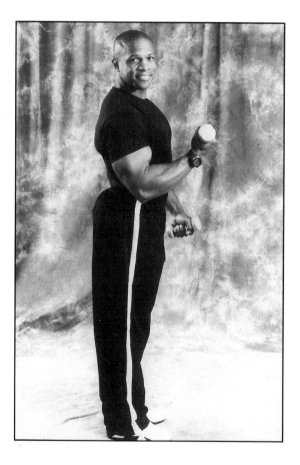

★     ★     ★

**Always consult your physician before starting
an exercise program.**

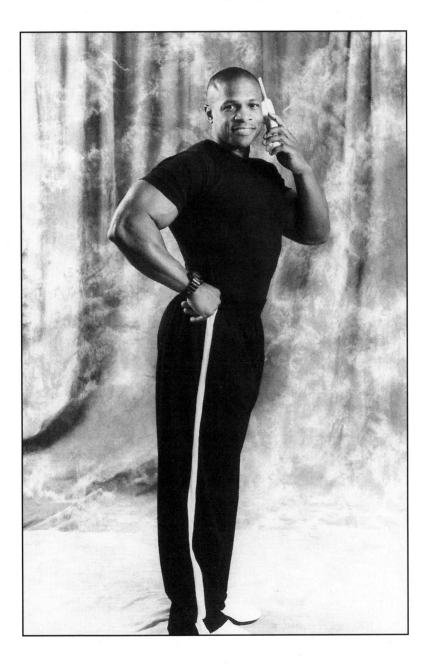

# FREQUENTLY USED TERMS

**Repetition:**
The completion of an exercise from start to finish.

**Set:**
A group of repetitions without rest.

**Correct breathing:**
Exhale on the exertion of the exercise.

**Rest:**
Rest is pause between exercises. Rest for as long as it takes to start the next exercise.

**Program design:**
I recommend using this program two to three days a week on nonconsecutive days for maximum results.

**Workout:**
The exercises contained in this program.

**Weight:**
Refers to the resistance used during the exercise, for example the weight of hand weights.

**Progressive body-shaping:**
Periodically increasing the weight on a specific exercise, especially when the weight being used is no longer a challenge.

★ ★ ★

# BODYSHAPING

1

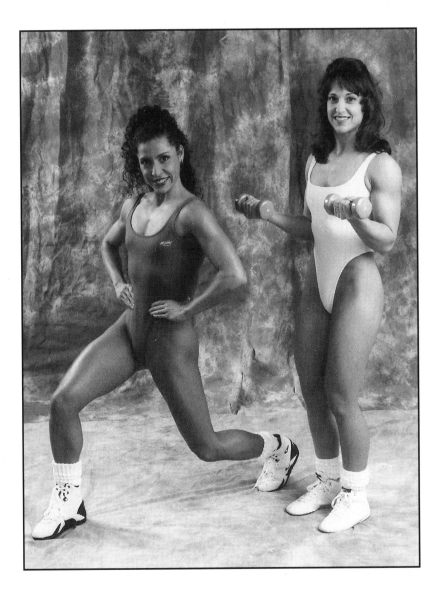

A ny woman can be as fit at fifty as she was
at twenty, providing she knows how to
train her body. My system is based on two
principles:

* Train the whole body;

* Try to exceed yourself every third workout to
  create progression.

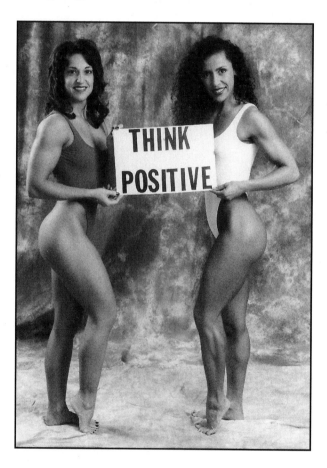

**THE FITNESS SYSTEM THAT NEVER FAILS**

# ALL YOU NEED IS
# A PAIR OF HAND WEIGHTS

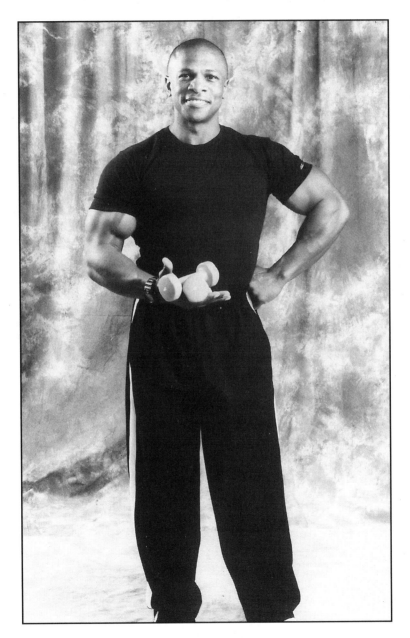

# THIS IS WHAT YOU CAN EXPECT!

**BEFORE**

**AFTER**

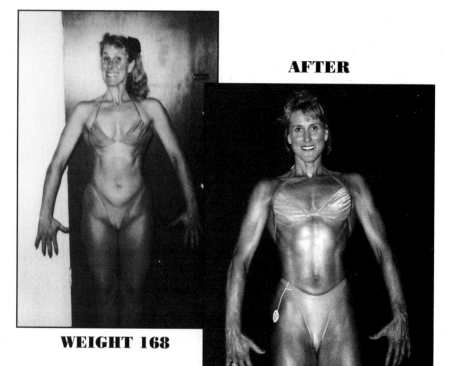

**WEIGHT 168**

**WEIGHT 138**

## DEBBIE RABALAIS

# THIS CAN BE YOU!

**BEFORE**

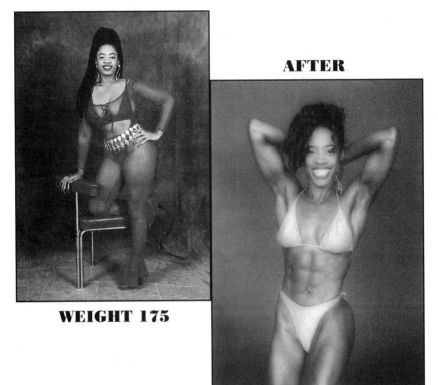

**AFTER**

**WEIGHT 175**

**WEIGHT 134**

# TREASHURE HOLLINGWORTH

# REMEMBER:

Your body will change whether you choose to change it or not. **You have the power to choose the direction.**

# DEBRA JACKSON

**BEFORE**

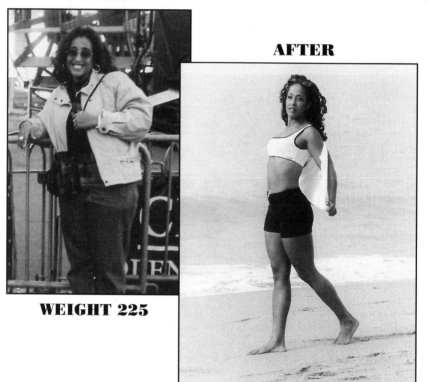

**AFTER**

**WEIGHT 225**

**WEIGHT 128**

# YOU CAN DO IT, TOO!

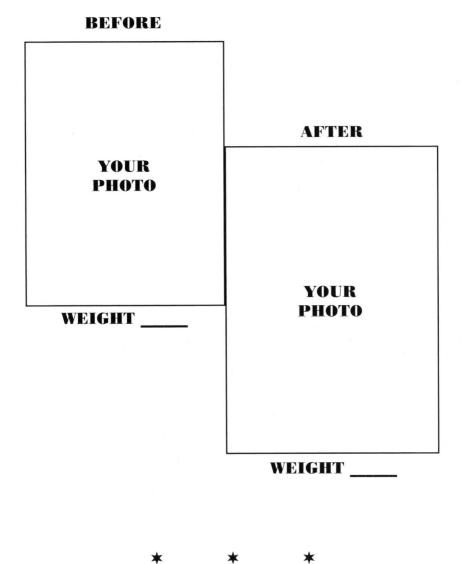

BEFORE

AFTER

YOUR
PHOTO

YOUR
PHOTO

WEIGHT _____

WEIGHT _____

★   ★   ★

# KEYS TO A BEAUTIFUL HEALTHY BODY

* A positive mental attitude

* A definite goal

* A plan to achieve your goal

* An unyielding belief that you can achieve your goal

* Take a step toward your goal every day

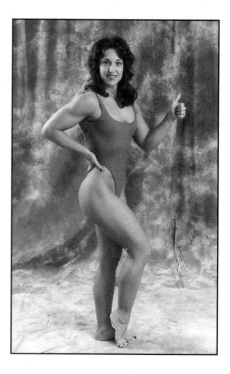

*"You are above all things, not below all things."*
~ *The Beautiful Woman*

★       ★       ★

Take a picture of yourself. You may not like what you see, but this will motivate you to exercise, make better food choices and make some lifestyle changes.

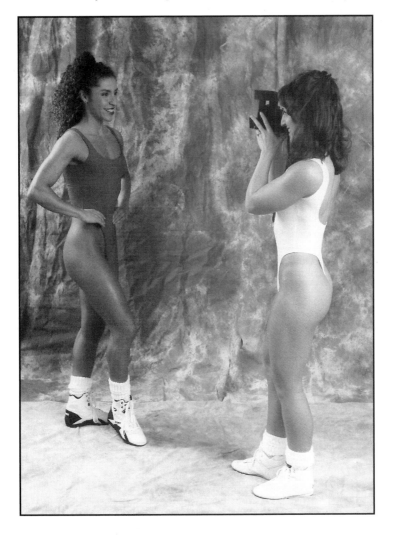

**To change your picture—you have to change your habits!**

# SELF IMAGE

List three things you like about yourself (for example):

1. I like my smile.
2. I like my attitude.
3. I like my legs.

List three reasons why regular exercise is important (for example):

1. Keeps my heart fit.
2. Keeps my muscles strong.
3. I feel great when I exercise.

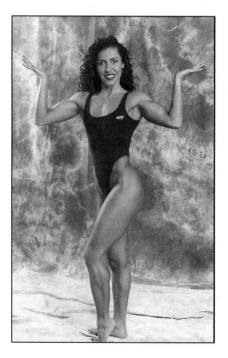

Where will you be, and how much will you weigh ten years from now, if you keep doing what you are doing today?

Write down your thoughts on a separate sheet of paper and start right now to change your direction.

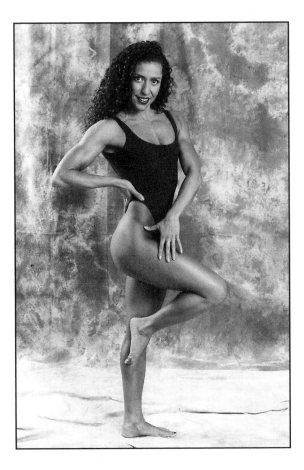

**Let your actions lead you
toward your goals.**

# 2

# BODYSHAPING BENEFITS

Just as aerobic exercise and balanced nutrition will help you lose fat, bodyshaping will improve posture, attitude, physical strength and reduce body fat. Bodyshaping will also increase muscle tone and enhance your natural curves. Bodyshaping uses resistance training (handweights) to shape your body by increasing muscle strength.

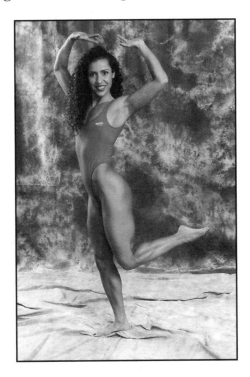

# THE BODYSHAPING SYSTEM

* Select starting weight
  Choose a light hand weight and focus on form and technique with each exercise.

* Repetitions
  Do twenty repetitions per exercise.

* If you can't do twenty repetitions per exercise, decrease starting weight one or two pounds.

* When you can easily do twenty repetitions per exercise, increase weight one or two pounds.

Progressive bodyshaping is a constant challenge. This is the key to a firm, tight, and healthy body.

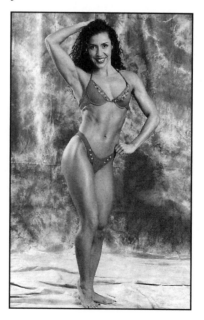

# THE BODYSHAPING PROCESS

* In the beginning you will experience brief periods of minor soreness.

* You will see yourself becoming more shapely.

* You will see regular increases in repetitions and strength on all exercises.

* You will automatically start setting higher fitness goals.

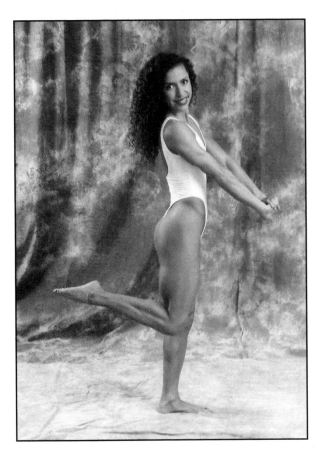

## QUICK GUIDELINES ON YOUR BODYSHAPING WORKOUT

* Don't skip the warm-up segment.
* Follow all exercise instructions.
* Don't rest between exercises.
* Remember to breathe.
* Think positive.

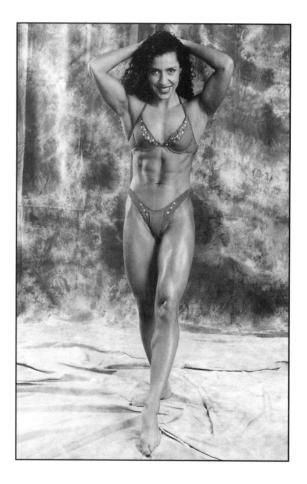

# SET FITNESS GOALS

Setting goals will help you change your body from the way it is now to the way you want it to be. It is important to set goals you can achieve. List your short-term and long-term goals for fat loss and fitness on a separate sheet of paper.

## Example:

**Short-term goals:** Lose one pound of fat a week, exercise three times a week and improve the quality of my nutrition.

**Long-term goals:** Lose 25 pounds of fat and make exercise and proper nutrition a part of my daily life style.

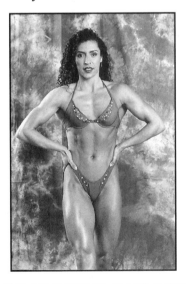

**SET GOALS YOU CAN ACHIEVE**

It is important to integrate your workout into your weekly schedule. This will aid you in following my program. To begin, select the days of the week you plan to exercise, the time of day, as well as the duration of each workout session. Be realistic!

Complete the chart at the bottom of this page before you start your workout.

## Example:
# PLAN YOUR WORKOUT

Exercise three days per week on nonconsecutive days.

Day 1:   MON

Day 2:   WED

Day 3:   FRI

Time of Day:   7:00 am

Duration of Each Workout (minutes):  12 min.

★　　★　　★

## Example:

# READ AND SIGN THIS AGREEMENT

I know that I can achieve my fitness goals. Therefore, I demand of myself persistence and continuous action toward its attainment daily.

Signature:   Robin Sandoval

Date:   July 21, 2000

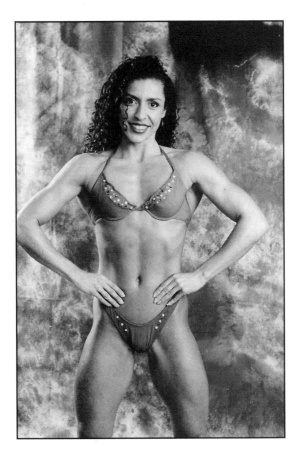

# Sample:
## WEEKLY EXERCISE RECORD
### Week of February 14 - 20, 2000

|  | Body-shaping | Weights | Aerobics exercise | Time | Notes |
|---|---|---|---|---|---|
| MON | **YES** | 3 pounds | Walking | 20 Min. | Good workout |
| TUES |  |  | REST DAY |  |  |
| WED | **YES** | 3 pounds | Walking | 20 Min. | Felt great |
| THUR |  |  | REST DAY |  |  |
| FRI | **YES** | 4 pounds | Walking | 20 Min. | I like it now |
| SAT | **NO** |  | Walking | 40 Min. | Slow pace |
| SUN |  |  | REST DAY |  |  |

## RECORD FOR SUCCESS

✱       ✱       ✱

# REMEMBER:

You cannot get in shape in one day, so don't try. Pace yourself. You will reach your goals.

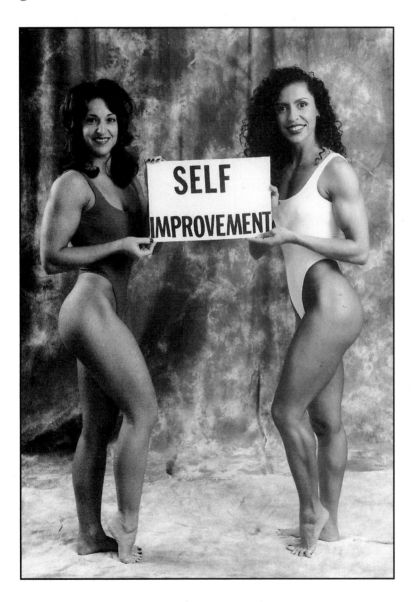

# THOUGHTS ON HEALTH AND FITNESS

* The more you repeat your goal, the greater your chance of achieving it.

* Remember, every piece of food you eat is either taking you toward or away from your goal.

* Focus your energy on one goal at a time.

* Don't let anything stop you.

* Turn all your negative thoughts about yourself into positive thoughts.

    I can go from unfit to fit.

    I can go from eating unhealthy to healthy.

    I am going to look and feel great.

    I expect positive lifestyle changes.

* Make up your mind to overcome every obstacle that is in front of you.

* Accept the priceless gift: the joy of exercise.

*     *     *

# THE BENEFITS OF EXERCISE

You are a mind with a body; therefore, mental fitness and physical fitness go hand-in-hand. Your attitude about exercise and proper nutrition must change from negative to positive in order to meet your fitness and fat loss goals.

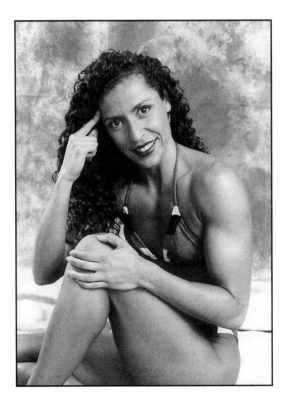

The mind is a complex recording system that can be programmed for success or failure. Program your mind for success by meditating on positive thoughts daily. How do you keep your mind positive so that you can achieve your goals?

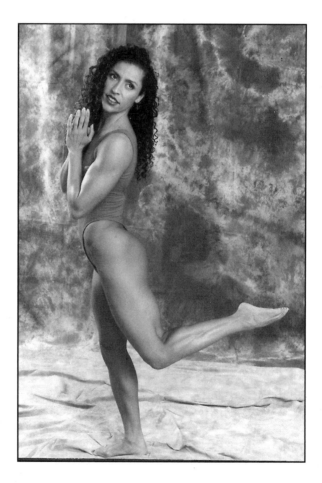

★　　　★　　　★

Renewing your mind every morning will guarantee your success. The Daily Mental Workout on the following pages will help you in this process.

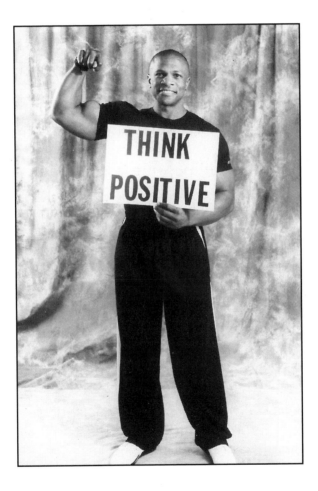

★　　　★　　　★

# DAILY MENTAL WORKOUT

The mind, like the body, needs daily exercise to be fit and healthy. Simply spending five minutes each day reading inspirational or motivational materials will fuel you daily as you pursue your goals. Start each day with an inspiring thought. The biggest secret of achievement is having a picture of a successful outcome in your mind.

* You were born to succeed.

* Pursue your goal as if you cannot fail.

* Your goal will become your reality.

* Repeat regularly: "I know I will achieve my goal."

* Set your goal and keep trying until you achieve it.

* Break big goals down into smaller ones.

* Focus on one weight loss at a time.

* Focus on the one reason you can achieve your goals, rather than the one hundred reasons you cannot.

* Do not focus on what you are going through. Focus instead on what you are going to look like when you reach your goal.

* Obstacles are those frightening things you see when you take your eyes off your goals.

* Believe that you are becoming healthier and healthier day by day.

* Whenever you want to eat unhealthy foods, stop, and repeat this:

**Eat healthy!   Eat healthy!   Eat healthy!**

Your desire for unhealthy foods will soon be replaced with a desire for healthy foods.

* You can be what you want to be if you are willing to pay the price.

The days that you skip your daily mental workout are probably the days you will have a tough time sticking to your program. If you read the thought conditioners every day, you will achieve your goals more easily.

*       *       *

# REMEMBER:

Every morning, take sixty seconds and visualize yourself succeeding at your body-shaping, nutrition and chosen aerobic activity for the day. This will provide you with a daily mental success plan.

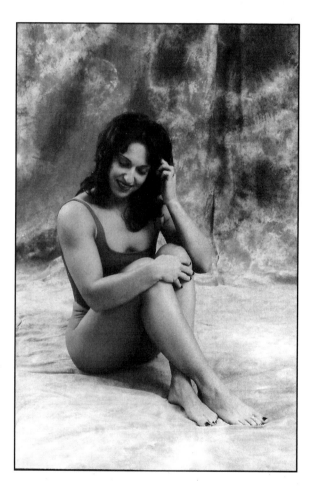

★　　★　　★

# THE BENEFITS OF EXERCISE...
## MENTAL

* Positive mental attitude
* Clearer thinking
* Happy moods
* Improved self image and self esteem
* Improved body image and appearance
* Improved outlook on life and sense of well being
* Special feeling of accomplishment
* Improved quality of your life
* You will feel wonderful!

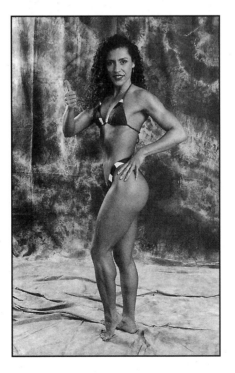

# BENEFITS OF EXERCISE...
# MEDICAL

Let there be no misunderstanding! Your health is one of your most valuable assets. Many people would be willing to trade their wealth for good health. The physiological benefits of exercise include:

* Decreased risk of heart disease
* Decrease in high blood pressure
* Decreased cholesterol levels
* Decreased triglycerides
* Decreased risk of obesity
* Decreased low density lipoproteins (LDL)
* Anxiety prevention
* Increased tolerance to stress
* Increased high density lipoproteins (HDL)
* Improvement in the quality of life

These benefits should be enough to get you to exercise now and keep you exercising for a lifetime.

*       *       *

# THE BENEFITS OF EXERCISE...
## PHYSICAL

* Stronger heart
* Increased endurance
* Increased muscle shape and tone
* Stronger bones
* Thinner body
* Increased flexi-bility
* Increased calorie burning
* Increased physical strength

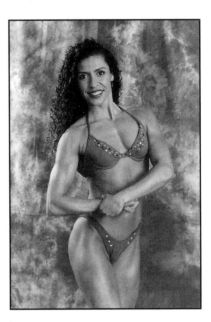

* Injury prevention
* Decreased body fat
* Decreased resting heart rate
* Improved sex life

\*     \*     \*

As you exercise, your body fat will decrease and your new shape and tone will hold everything in place in a most pleasing way.

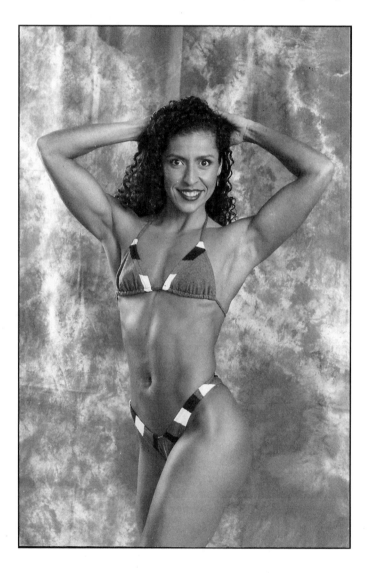

## SEE WHAT CAN HAPPEN?

\*     \*     \*

# ANATOMY CHARTS

# FRONT
# AND
# BACK

\*     \*     \*

# ANATOMY CHART
# (FRONT)

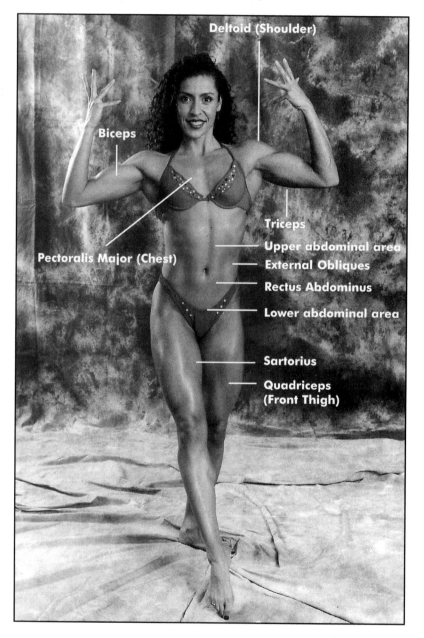

Deltoid (Shoulder)

Biceps

Triceps

Upper abdominal area

External Obliques

Pectoralis Major (Chest)

Rectus Abdominus

Lower abdominal area

Sartorius

Quadriceps
(Front Thigh)

# ANATOMY CHART
# (BACK)

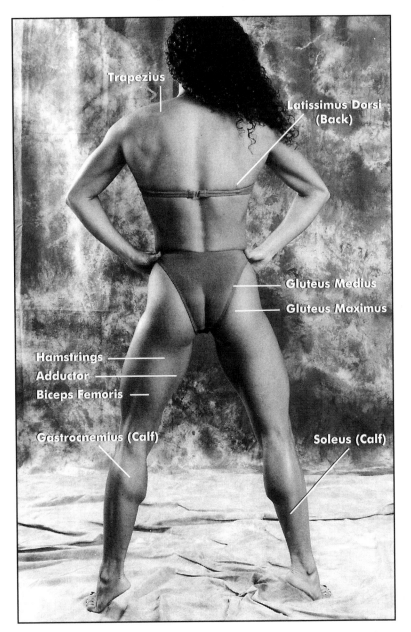

Trapezius

Latissimus Dorsi
(Back)

Gluteus Medius

Gluteus Maximus

Hamstrings

Adductor

Biceps Femoris

Gastrocnemius (Calf)

Soleus (Calf)

# KEYS TO KEEPING IT GOING

* Plan regular exercise

* Keep track of your progress

* Measure your improvements

* Evaluate and redefine your goals as you progress

* Look in the mirror and note the changes

* Exercise with a friend

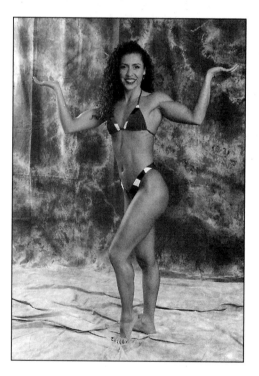

## KEEP A GOAL IN FRONT OF YOU

# THE UPPER BODY WORKOUT

**4**

## NOW ITS TIME TO SHAPE AND TONE THE UPPER BODY

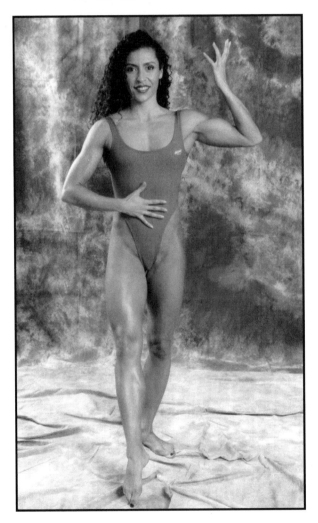

# Warm Up (Marching in Place)

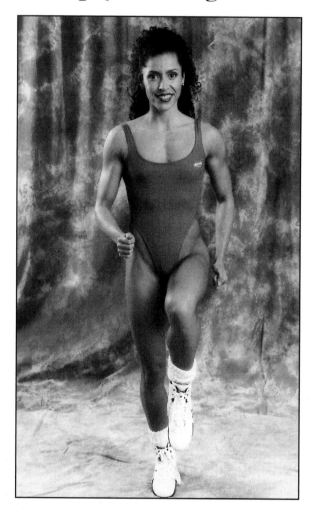

## 5 MINUTES

&#9733;   &#9733;   &#9733;

# YOU DESERVE IT!
# LET'S GET BUSY

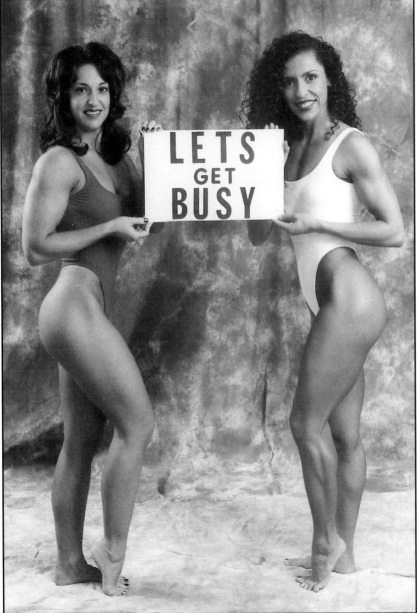

# CHEST

## BENCH PRESS WITH HAND WEIGHTS

This exercise will shape and tone the chest, shoulders and triceps.

**Position:**
Lie flat on the floor with your knees bent. Arch your chest upward, holding weights on either side of your chest.

**Movement:**
Keep your body stable and slowly press the weights to the straight arm position, pause briefly and repeat.

**Breathing:**
Exhale as you press upward.

**Goal:**
Twenty repetitions.

★     ★     ★

# BENCH PRESS WITH HAND WEIGHTS

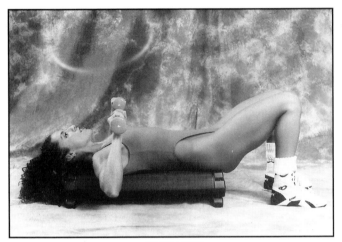

**START**

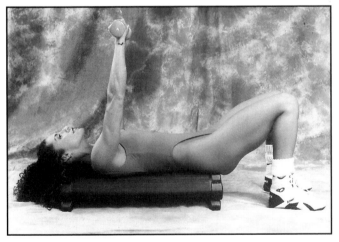

**FINISH**

## 20 REPETITIONS

### No resting. Move to the next exercise.

# BACK

## REVERSE ROWS WITH HAND WEIGHTS

This exercise will shape and tone your back and biceps.

**Position:**
Shoulder-width stance. Put a slight bend in your knees, bend over with your back flat and extend arms with weights.

**Movement:**
Keep your body stable. Pull the weights to your chest, pause briefly, and slowly lower to the starting position.

**Breathing:**
Exhale as you pull the weights to your chest.

**Goal:**
Twenty repetitions.

★　　★　　★

# REVERSE ROWS WITH
# HAND WEIGHTS

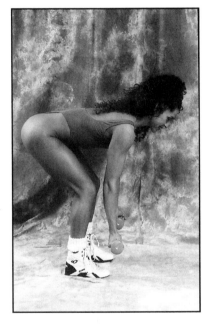 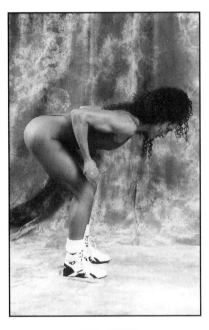

**START**                    **FINISH**

## 20 REPETITIONS

### No resting. Move to the next exercise.

# SHOULDERS

## SHOULDER PRESS WITH HAND WEIGHTS

This exercise will shape and tone your shoulders and the back of the upper arm.

**Position:**
Feet should be shoulder-width apart. Put a slight bend in your knees and keep your back flat. Hold your chest high with weights on the side of your shoulders.

**Movement:**
Keep your body stable, with weights on the side of your shoulders. Press them straight up, pause briefly, and slowly lower to the starting position.

**Breathing:**
Exhale as you press upward.

**Goal:**
Twenty repetitions.

★       ★       ★

# SHOULDER PRESS WITH
# HAND WEIGHTS

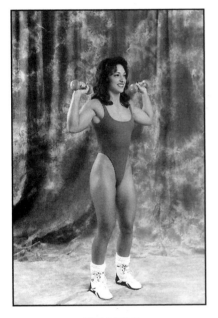

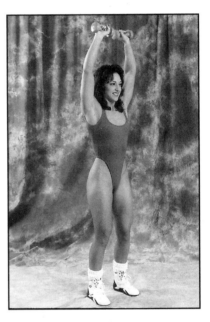

**START**          **FINISH**

## 20 REPETITIONS
### No resting. Move to next exercise.

# BICEPS

## CURLS WITH HAND WEIGHTS

This exercise will shape and tone the front of your arms.

**Position:**
Shoulder-width stance. Put a slight bend in your knees and keep your back flat and chest high with weights at your side.

**Movement:**
Keeping your body stable, curl the weights to your shoulders. Pause briefly, and slowly lower to the starting position.

**Breathing:**
Exhale as you bend your arms.

**Goal:**
Twenty repetitions..

★      ★      ★

# CURLS WITH HAND WEIGHTS

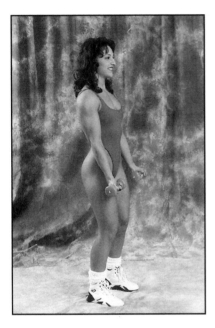

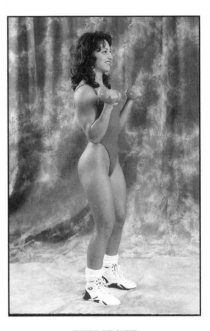

**START**
          **FINISH**

## 20 REPETITIONS
No resting. Move to next exercise.

# TRICEPS

## STANDING FRENCH PRESS

This exercise will shape and tone the back of the upper arms.

**Position:**
Shoulder-width stance. Put a slight bend in your knees and keep your back flat and chest high. With both hands, hold a hand weight behind your head.

**Movement:**
Keep your body stable. Holding the weight, slowly extend your arms overhead. Keeping the elbows high, slowly lower the weight to the starting position behind the neck. Pause briefly, and repeat.

**Breathing:**
Exhale as you press upward.

**Goal:**
Twenty repetitions.

★    ★    ★

# STANDING FRENCH PRESS

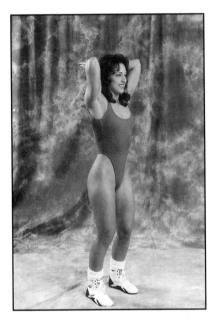

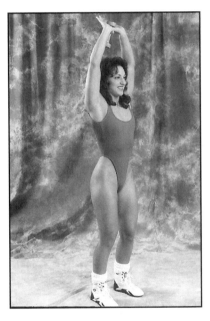

**START**

**FINISH**

## 20 REPETITIONS
### No resting. Move to the next exercise.

Don't stop now. You're doing great! Repeat the following affirmations:

I feel healthy!

I feel happy!

I feel terrific!

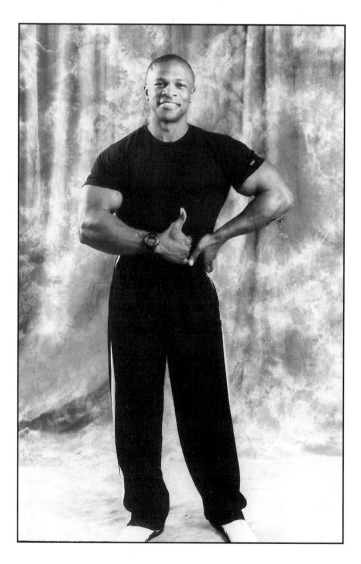

# THOUGHTS ON HEALTH AND FITNESS

* A positive attitude is your passport to a healthier tomorrow.

* Expect to succeed.

* To be physically fit you must first be mentally fit.

* Stick to your program regardless of the difficulties you are bound to experience.

* Exercise is the lubricant that keeps the human body running evenly and smoothly.

* Cultivate the friendship of those who have confidence in your ability to succeed.

* Avoid people who are negative or who put you down.

* Laughter aids digestion.

* Acquiring a long-term problem in exchange for short-term pleasure is not a good bargain.

* Wishing never got anybody anything. Don't wish; take action.

*      *      *

# 5

# THE LOWER BODY WORKOUT

It's time to shape and tone the lower body. Don't you love it?

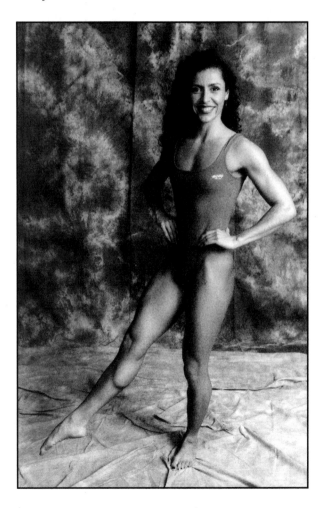

# CALVES

## CALF RAISE WITH HAND WEIGHTS

This exercise will shape and tone the back of the lower leg.

**Position:**
Standing with your feet shoulder-width apart, put a slight bend in your knees and keep your back flat and chest high while holding weights at the side of your thighs.

**Movement:**
Keep your body stable, slowly rise onto the toes, pause briefly, and return heels to floor.

**Breathing:**
Exhale as you go up on your toes.

**Goal:**
Twenty repetitions.

✴     ✴     ✴

# CALF RAISE WITH HAND WEIGHTS

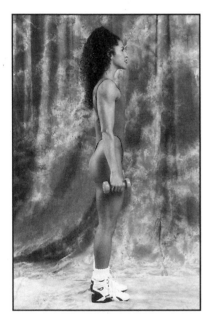

**START**

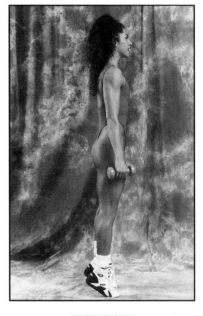

**FINISH**

## 20 REPETITIONS
**No resting. Move to next exercise.**

# THIGHS

## SQUATS WITH HAND WEIGHTS

This exercise will shape and tone the front of the thighs and buttocks.

**Position:**
Standing with feet shoulder-width apart, put a slight bend in your knees and keep your back flat. Your chest should be high while holding weights at the side of your thighs.

**Movement:**
Keep your torso stable and slowly lower your body until your thighs are parallel to the floor. Rising to a standing position, pause briefly, and repeat.

**Breathing:**
Exhale as your straighten your legs.

**Goal:**
Twenty repetitions.

★　　　★　　　★

# SQUATS WITH HAND WEIGHTS

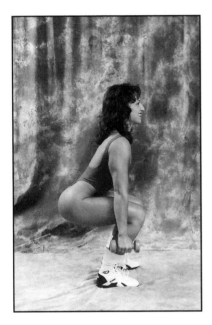 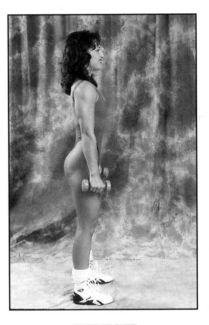

**START**  **FINISH**

## 20 REPETITIONS
### No resting. Move to the next exercise.

# THIGHS

## FRONT SQUATS WITH HAND WEIGHT

This exercise will shape and tone the front of the thighs.

**Position:**
Standing with feet shoulder-width apart, put a slight bend in your knees and keep your back flat and chest high, with weight held on your upper chest.

**Movement:**
Keep your torso stable, slowly lower your body until your thighs are parallel to the floor, then rise to a standing position, pause briefly and repeat.

**Breathing:**
Exhale as you straighten your legs.

**Goal:**
Twenty repetitions.

★　　　★　　　★

# FRONT SQUATS WITH
# HAND WEIGHT

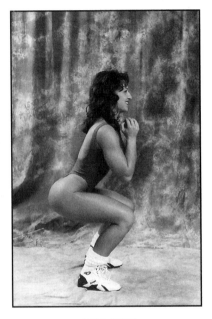

**START**

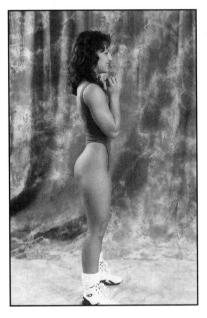

**FINISH**

## 20 REPETITIONS
### No resting. Move to the next exercise.

# THIGHS AND BUTTOCKS

## LUNGES WITH HAND WEIGHTS

This exercise will shape and tone your thighs and buttocks.

**Position:**
Standing with feet shoulder-width apart, put a slight bend in your knees and keep your back flat and chest high, with weights at the side of your thighs.

**Movement:**
Keep your torso stable and take a long step forward with one foot and bend the knee to a fencer's lunge position. Push back to a standing position, pause briefly, and repeat exercise with the other leg.

**Breathing:**
Exhale as you return to the standing position.

**Goal:**
Forty repetitions.

★    ★    ★

# LUNGES WITH HAND WEIGHTS

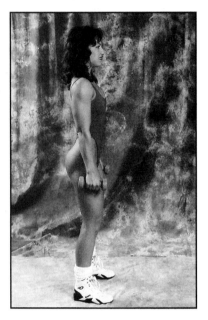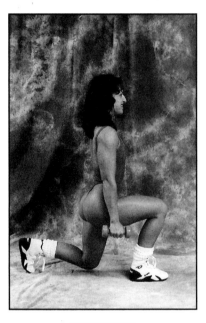

**START**                    **FINISH**

## 40 REPETITIONS
### No resting. Move to the next exercise.

# HAMSTRINGS

## LEG CURLS WITH HAND WEIGHT

This exercise will shape and tone the back of your upper thighs.

**Position:**
Lie flat on the floor with a weight between your feet and keep a slight bend in your knees.

**Movement:**
Keep your body stable and pull your lower leg to your body. Pause briefly and lower to the starting position.

**Breathing:**
Exhale as you bend your lower leg.

**Goal:**
Twenty repetitions.

★      ★      ★

# LEG CURLS WITH HAND WEIGHT

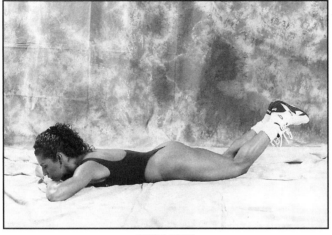

**START**

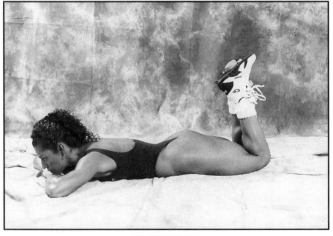

**FINISH**

## 20 REPETITIONS
### No resting. Move to the next exercise.

Great job! That was the end of your lower body workout. Whew!!!!

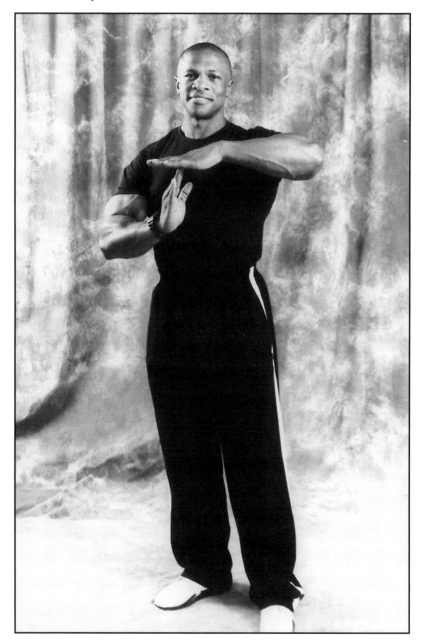

# THOUGHTS ON HEALTH AND FITNESS

* Keep your goal in mind, and it will become a reality.

* Goals are as essential to success as oxygen is to life.

* Always have a new goal.

* Unhappiness is the greatest cause of sickness and disease. Stay happy and stay healthy.

* To remain young, take care of how you live in your thought world.

* Exercise is one of the secrets for dodging old age.

* Good habits are as easy to form as bad ones.

* Stop putting yourself down.

* Don't let yourself be pushed around by past events.

* When it comes to eating, you can sometimes help yourself more by helping yourself to less.

* To start the day with a prayer is to start the day with a song.

*     *     *

# THE ABBOMINALS 6

Your waistline dictates your life line: the smaller the waistline, the longer the life line. Now let's shape and tone the abdominal area.

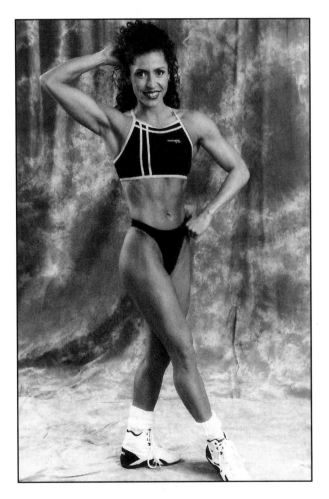

# LOWER ABDOMINALS

## ALTERNATE KNEE-INS

This exercise will shape, tone and tighten the lower and upper abdominal area.

**Position:**
Lie on the floor with your legs slightly bent in front of you. Place the palms of your hand flat on the floor and under your lower back.

**Movement:**
From the starting position, alternate your knees in and out toward your chest in a bicycle-like movement. Pause briefly on each repetition.

**Breathing:**
Exhale as you bring your knees to your chest.

**Goal:**
Forty repetitions.

✱    ✱    ✱

# ALTERNATE KNEE-INS

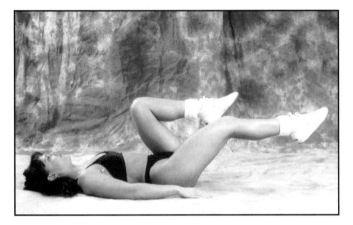

**START**

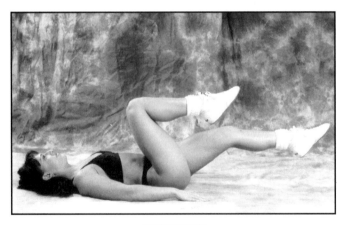

**FINISH**

## 40 REPETITIONS
**No resting. Move to the next exercise.**

# ABDOMINALS
# (EXTERNAL OBLIQUES)

## ALTERNATE TWISTING KNEE-INS

This exercise will shape and tone obliques and lower abdominal area.

**Position:**
Lie on your back on the floor and place your hand behind your head, knees bent and feet flat on the floor.

**Movement:**
Lying face up with the knees bent and the hands loosely placed along the side of your head, bring the opposite elbow and knee together. Pause briefly and alternate with each repetition.

**Breathing:**
Exhale as elbows and knees come together.

**Goal:**
Forty repetitions.

\*　　　\*　　　\*

# ALTERNATE TWISTING KNEE-INS

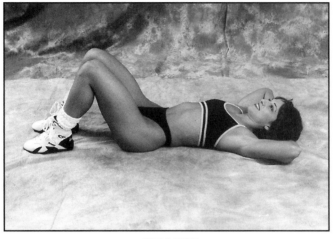

**START**

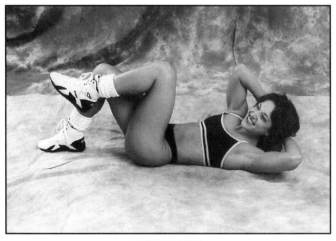

**FINISH**

## 40 REPETITIONS

**No resting. Move to the next exercise.**

# ABDOMINALS
# (UPPER AND LOWER)

## KNEE-RAISED CRUNCHES

This exercise will shape and tone the upper and lower abdominal area.

**Position:**
Lie flat on your back on the floor and pull both knees up until your legs form an 'L" position. Place your hands behind your head.

**Movement:**
Slowly curl the upper back off the floor while pressing the lower back against the floor. Pause briefly and repeat.

**Breathing:**
Exhale as you curl up.

**Goal:**
Forty repetitions.

*     *     *

# KNEE-RAISED CRUNCH

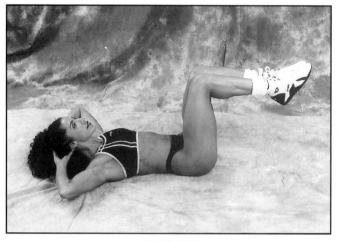

**START**

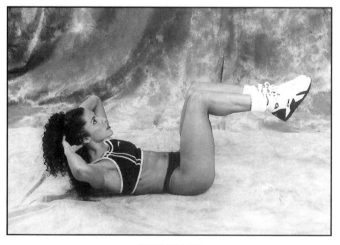

**FINISH**

## 40 REPETITIONS
**No resting. Move to the next exercise.**

T hat was our last exercise for the abdominals.

**Don't your abs feel great?
What a feeling!**

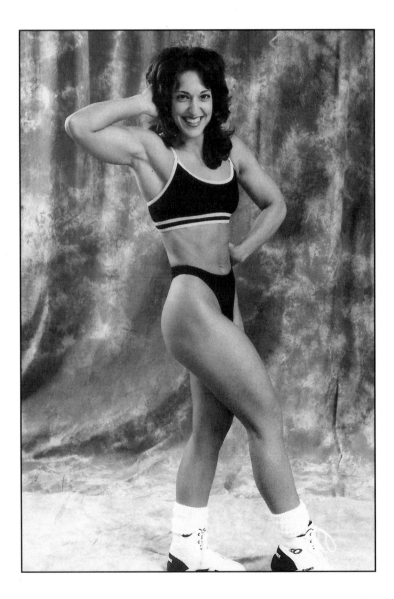

# THOUGHTS ON HEALTH AND FITNESS

* Remember, anyone can quit. That's the easy way out.

* There are no shortcuts to any place worth going.

* Replace "I can't" with "I can."

* Once you have overcome the crippling "I can't" block, there's no limit to what you can achieve.

* Remember, regardless of what you have been or what you are now, you can be what you want to be if you act with a positive mental attitude.

* Successful people have one thing in common: every time they fail, they try again.

* No matter how many dark clouds appear, the sun will shine again.

* Ask your creator to renew your strength, so you can "run, and not be weary...walk, and not faint."

* You cannot control the wind, but you can adjust your sail.

* No pessimist ever won a battle.

* Get the pollution of negative thinking out of your mind.

✱    ✱    ✱

# COOL DOWN AND STRETCH $^7$

Y ou just made a great investment in your
health and fitness.

Now it's time to cool down and stretch.

Give yourself a pat on the back!

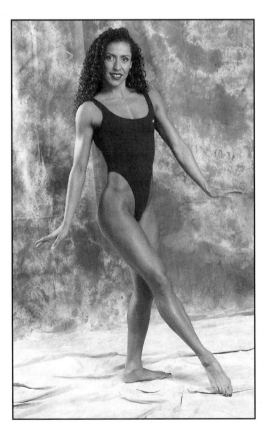

## THINGS TO REMEMBER
## WHILE STRETCHING

* Stretch when your body is warm. Never stretch a cold muscle.

* Stretch slowly and gently to the point of mild tension, not pain.

* Never bounce when stretching.

* Hold each stretch for ten seconds.

* Breathe slowly and deeply as you stretch. Don't hold your breath.

* Avoid locking your joints while stretching.

* Listen to your body and stretch within your limits.

*     *     *

# BASIC STRETCHES

## SHOULDER ROLLS

Keeping shoulders and arms relaxed, roll shoulders up and down. Repeat several times. This stretch increases flexibility of the shoulder joint and reduces tension in the neck and shoulder area.

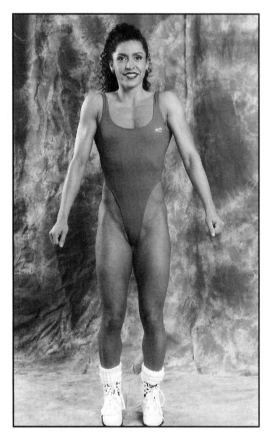

## REPEAT THREE TIMES

# CHEST STRETCH

Stand with feet shoulders width apart and knees relaxed. Hold chest up and shoulders back. Grasp hands behind your back. Keeping elbows slightly bent, squeeze shoulder blades together and gently lift arms until you feel a stretch across the chest and in the front of the shoulders. This exercise stretches out the chest.

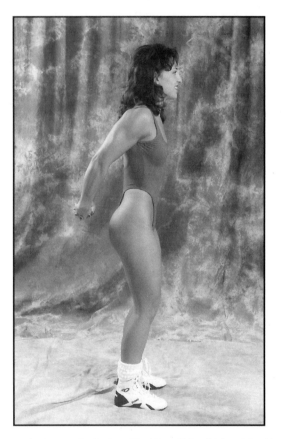

## HOLD FOR TEN SECONDS

# DELTOID STRETCH

Stand with feet shoulders width apart and knees relaxed. Hold chest up and shoulders back. Put one arm across the chest and pull toward the opposite shoulder with the other arm. Repeat for the other side. This exercise stretches out the shoulders.

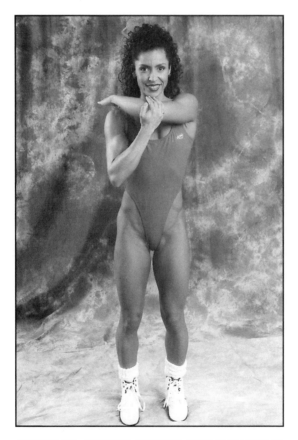

## HOLD FOR TEN SECONDS

# UPPER BACK STRETCH

Stand with feet shoulders width apart and knees slightly bent. Grasp hands with palms facing outward. Extend arms forward at shoulder height. Tuck your chin, and round your shoulders and upper back. This exercise stretches the upper back and upper arms.

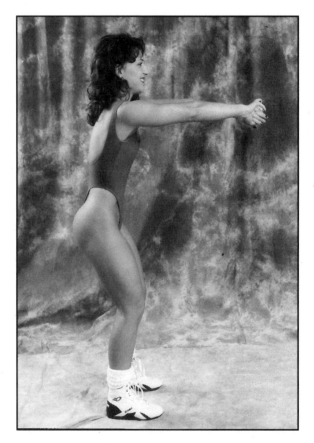

## HOLD FOR TEN SECONDS

# CALF STRETCH

Stand in a lunge position with toes straight ahead, both hands on the upper thigh of the lunging leg and heels flat on the floor. Bend the front knee and lean forward from the hips until you feel a stretch in the calf muscles of the rear leg. Repeat for the other leg. This exercise stretches the calf muscles.

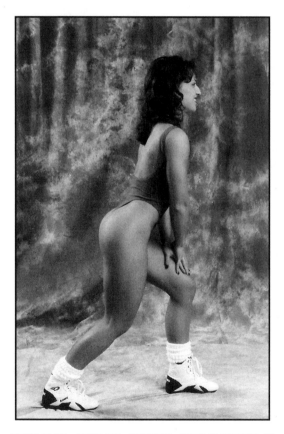

## HOLD FOR TEN SECONDS

# QUADRICEPS STRETCH
# (FRONT OF THIGH)

In a standing position, grasp the outside of the ankle with your hand. Gently pull foot toward your buttocks, making sure the knee is pointing straight down. Repeat for the other side. This exercise stretches the front of the thighs.

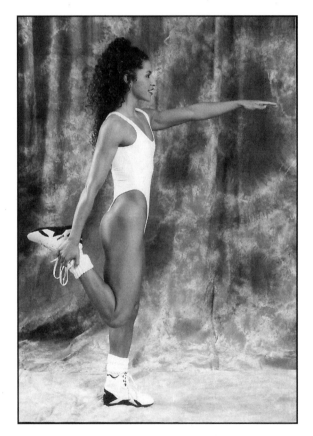

## HOLD FOR TEN SECONDS

# HIP ADDUCTORS STRETCH
# (INNER THIGHS)

Sit with soles of feet together, hands on ankles. Keeping rib cage lifted and head up, bend forward in the hips until you feel the stretch in the groin area. This exercise stretches the inner thighs.

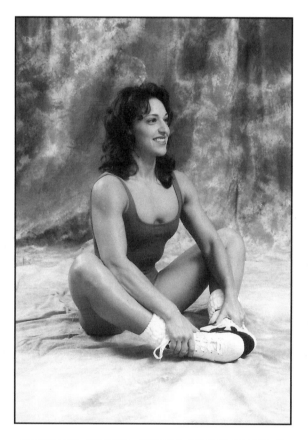

## HOLD FOR TEN SECONDS

# SPINAL TWIST

L ie on your back. Press your lower back down as you pull one knee into your chest keeping the other leg fully extended on the floor. Cross the bent knee over other leg, making sure both shoulders remain on the floor. Turn your head to look in the other direction. Repeat on the other side. This exercise stretches the lower back and side of hips.

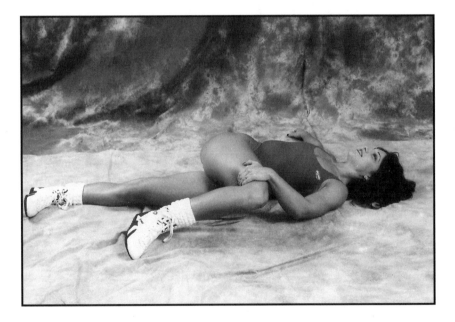

**HOLD FOR TEN SECONDS**

# HAMSTRING STRETCH

Lie on your back with one knee bent and the opposite leg extended straight upward. Grasp one leg below the knee and pull gently toward the chest. This exercise stretches the back of the leg.

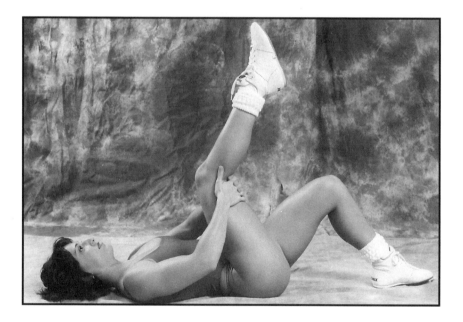

## HOLD FOR TEN SECONDS

# KNEE-TO-CHEST

L ie flat on your back with knees bent, feet on the floor. Pull both knees to your chest. This exercise stretches the lower back, buttocks and back of the thighs.

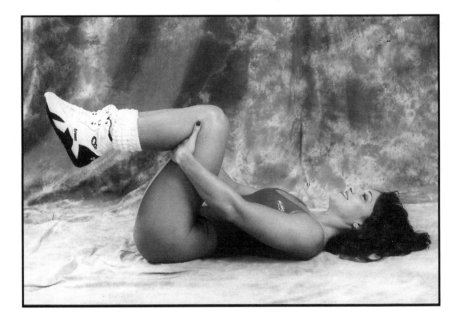

## HOLD FOR TEN SECONDS

# FULL BODY STRETCH

Lie flat on your back. Extend arms above your head and straighten legs. Point fingers and toes and stretch as far you can in opposite directions. This exercise stretches and relaxes the entire body.

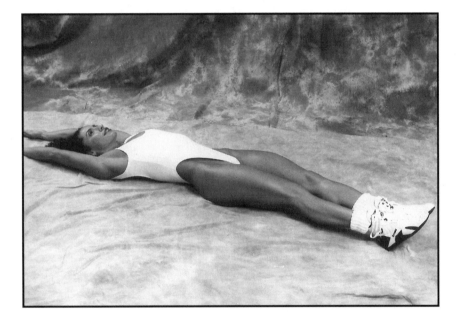

## HOLD FOR TEN SECONDS

# GREAT WORKOUT!

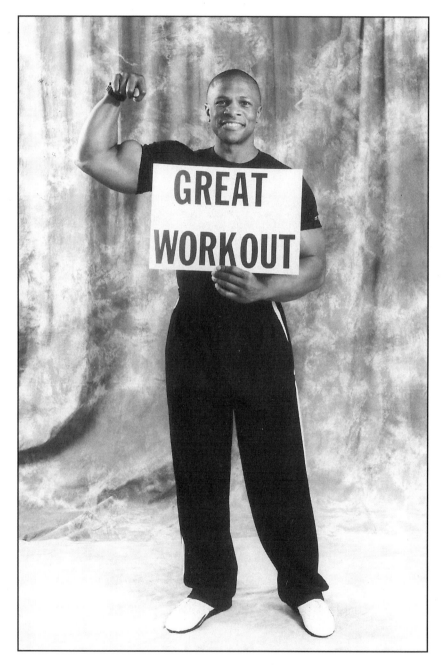

# THOUGHTS ON HEALTH AND FITNESS

* Focus on self improvement.

* No discipline, no improvement. It's simple!

* God did not create you to suffer defeat.

* Setbacks pave the way for comebacks.

* One of the secrets of a long and fruitful life is to forgive everybody, everything, every night, before you go to bed.

* Turn tragedy into triumph.

* It is better to wear out than to rust out.

* No matter how far you fall, you are never out of God's reach.

* It's not the size of the dog in the fight that counts, but the size of the fight in the dog.

* Every good and perfect gift is from above.

* God is my strength and power. God makes my way perfect.

★     ★     ★

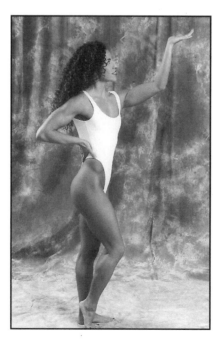

# BENEFITS OF AEROBICS

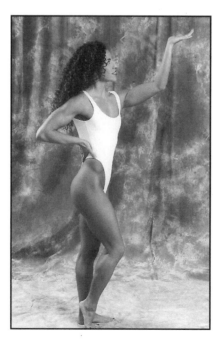

If you are five to eight pounds above your ideal weight or even if you need to shed an extra thirty to forty pounds, aerobic exercise is the ticket. Additional benefits of aerobics include:

* Increased life expectancy
* Enhanced feeling of well being
* Increased lean muscle mass

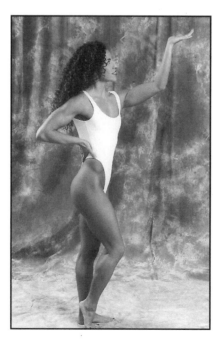

# AEROBIC EXERCISE

Aerobic exercise will get your heart and lungs in shape and reduce unwanted body fat. Your aerobic exercise plan should incorporate the following:

* **Frequency:** Three times per week

* **Intensity:** Once your exercise becomes easy, increase your speed to increase the intensity.

* **Duration:** Fifteen to thirty minutes per session.

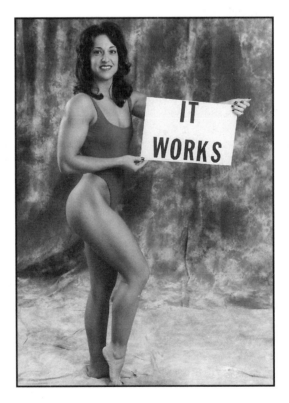

# THINGS TO REMEMBER

* Proper foot wear is very important.

* Always warm-up and cool down.

* Gradually increase duration.

* Gradually increase pace or speed only after you have achieved your duration.

* If you cannot talk while exercising, you are working too hard.

* Keep a record of daily exercises.

* Track your progress; that is, time your walks.

* Plan your workout in advance.

* Avoid setting unreasonable goals.

*   *   *

# AEROBICS

## LIFECYCLE

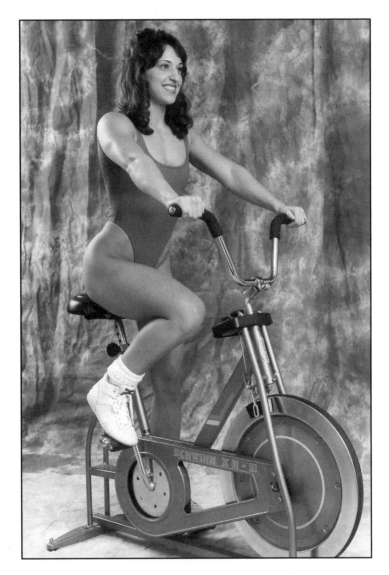

## SAFE AND EFFECTIVE
## FAT BURNING EXERCISE

# AEROBICS
## WALKING

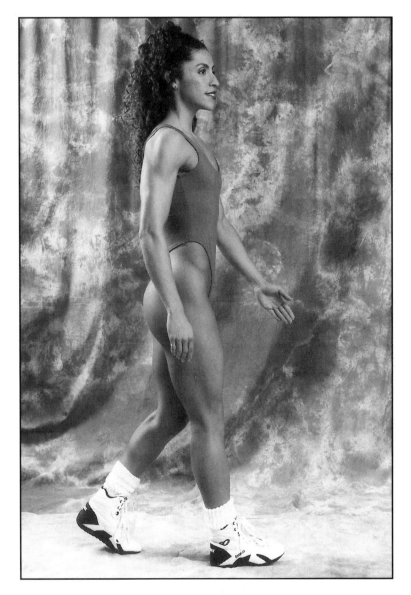

**KEEP YOUR CHEST AND HEAD HIGH!**

# AEROBICS

## POWERWALKING

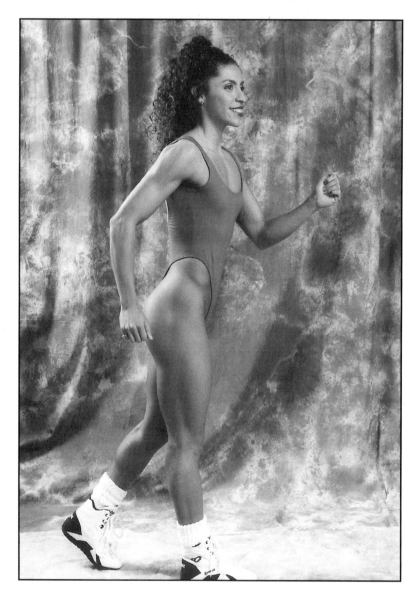

## HEEL-TO-TOE WALKING

# WALKING PROGRAM

* **WEEK 1**
  Walk ten minutes daily.

* **WEEK 2**
  Walk fifteen minutes daily.

* **WEEK 3**
  Walk twenty minutes daily.

* **WEEK 4**
  Walk twenty-five minutes daily.

* **WEEK 5**
  Walk thirty minutes daily.

* **WEEK 6**
  Set your own daily walking goal. On a separate sheet of paper write down how many minutes you plan to walk daily.

### YOU ARE THE CAPTAIN OF THE SHIP

*       *       *

# THOUGHTS ON HEALTH AND FITNESS

* Stay with it!

* What you get when you achieve your goals is not nearly as important as what you become when you reach them.

* It's always too soon to quit.

* You are bigger and tougher than any obstacle you will ever face.

* You are invincible.

* Empty your mind of all negative thoughts.

* You can change just about anything in your life if you turn your life over to God.

* Cast your burden on the Lord and he will sustain you.

* Remember all the good things God has done for you in the past.

* Visualize all the good things God will do for you in the future.

* God's help is always available. Just ask.

*     *     *

# BACK CARE

Many back problems are due to one of the following:

* Poor lifting habits

* Tension and muscle tightness

* Poor posture

* Obesity

* Inactivity

* Lack of abdominal strength

* Tightened muscles in the lower back

* Tight hamstrings

On the next several pages, I will show you some things you can do to save your back.

\* \* \*

# CORRECT POSTURE

From the side view, a straight line should pass through your body. The head should be centered over the trunk and the shoulders should be down, and back, but relaxed. The chest should be high and the abdomen flat.

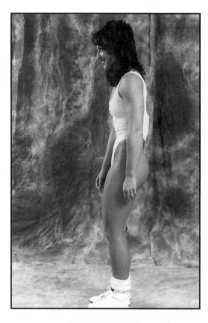 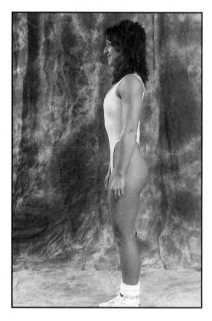

**WRONG**             **RIGHT**

## NOW STRAIGHTEN UP!

# LIFTING

Never lift anything with your legs straight. Always bend your knees when lifting.

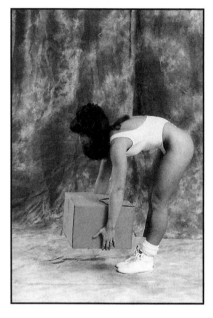

**WRONG**

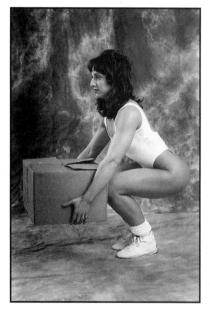

**RIGHT**

★　　★　　★

# SITTING

Never sit with your head and shoulders rounded forward. Keep your shoulders back and your back flat.

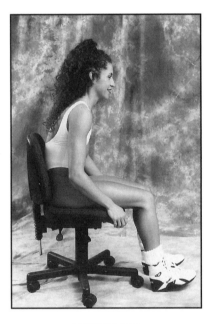

**WRONG**

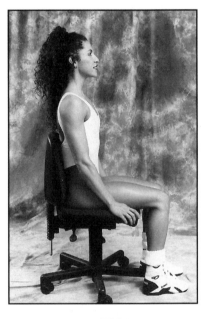

**RIGHT**

★      ★      ★

# PROLONGED STANDING

Prop one foot up on a box or stool to relieve back tension that comes from prolonged standing.

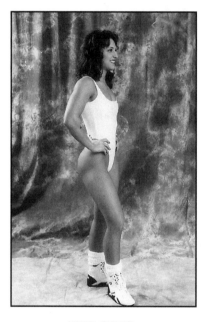

**WRONG**

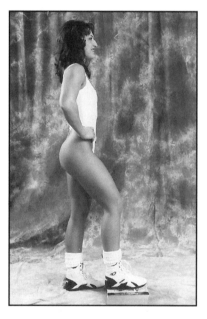

**RIGHT**

★　　★　　★

# SLEEPING OR LYING

Keep knees and hips bent to avoid lower back pain while you are sleeping or lying down.

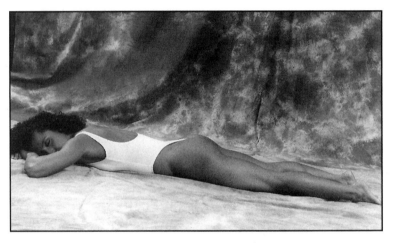

**WRONG**

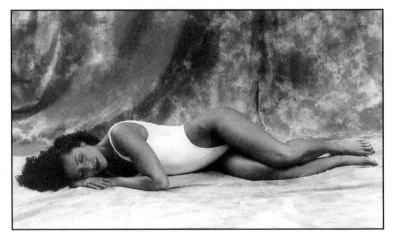

**RIGHT**

# THOUGHTS ON HEALTH AND FITNESS

* This is the day the Lord has made and I will rejoice and be glad in it.

* Expect the best and get the best.

* I believe I will successfully handle any problem that arises today.

* I can overcome any obstacle.

* God is with me and helping me.

* God will see me through this situation.

* I don't believe in defeat.

* A positive mind always delivers power.

* Difficulty is only mental.

* Faith always overcomes fear.

\*        \*        \*

# NUTRITION

# 10

Now that you have exercised your body, it's time to feed it properly. YOU ARE WHAT YOU EAT. Food builds your body. You have to eat lean to look lean, so build your body with the best foods.

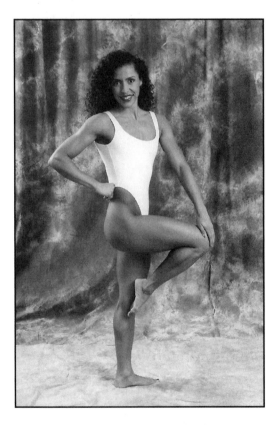

**YOU DESERVE THE BEST!**

# CHOICES

The key to proper nutrition is making the right choices. Eat fat and you become fat. Eat lean and you become lean. The choice is yours.

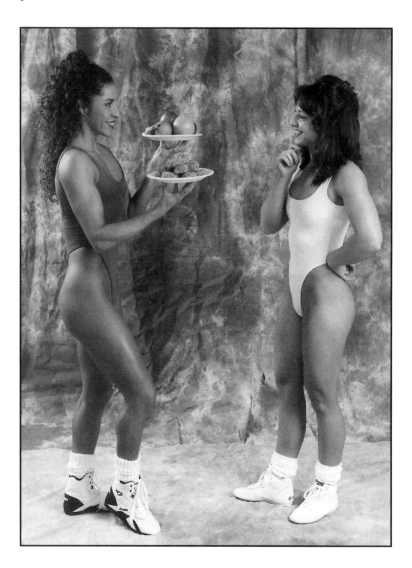

# THE PROPER WAY TO FUEL YOUR BODY

* Eat a variety of healthy foods daily.

* Avoid too much fat.

* If you drink coffee, tea or soda, do so in moderation.

* Eat slowly.

* Eat all meals at the table.

* Prepare small portions.

* Trim the excess fat on meats.

* Bake or broil rather than fry.

* Limit alcohol.

* Avoid late and heavy meals.

**"Your body is like your car.
Put the best gas in it."**

*        *        *

# NUTRIENTS AND THEIR JOBS

**Protein** contains amino acids. It builds and repairs muscle tissue. One gram of protein equals four calories.

**Carbohydrates** provide energy for the body. Good sources include grains, rice, potatoes and beans. One gram equals four calories.

**Fats** provide energy, energy storage, and insulation for the body. One gram equals nine calories. Fats are either monounsaturated, polyunsaturated, or saturated. Saturated fats come mainly from animal sources (meats and dairy products). They inhibit the removal of cholesterol from the blood. Saturated fats are solid at room temperature and are considered the "bad fat" in our diets.

**Polyunsaturated fats** come from plant sources and are liquid at room temperature. They help to lower the cholesterol in the blood and are considered the "good fat" in our diets. Monounsaturated fats are also considered to be "good fats." They are found in peanuts, canola, and olive oils. Like polyunsaturated fats, they are liquid at room temperature.

**Minerals** are organic substances needed in the diet in small amounts to help regulate bodily functions. Minerals do not provide calories, therefore, can't be used for energy.

**Vitamins** are organic compounds that function as metabolic regulators in the body. Vitamins are classified as water soluble or fat soluble. They do not have calories, therefore, cannot be used for energy.

**Water**, the most important nutrient, transports nutrients to cells and removes waste from cells and helps regulate body temperature.

★    ★    ★

# NUTRITIONAL DO'S AND DONT'S

| DO | DON'T |
| --- | --- |
| Reduce fat intake | Don't buy high fat foods |
| Slow down eating pace | Don't eat high fat foods |
| Take a bite every thirty seconds | Don't eat skin on meats |
| | Don't eat fried foods |
| Drink eight to ten glasses of water a day | Don't use sugar in your diet |
| Eat meals at regularly scheduled times | Don't use too much sodium |
| Bake, broil or grill meats | Don't eat ready-to-eat foods |
| Keep a nutrition journal | |
| Make a list before shopping for groceries | Don't be discouraged by occasional set backs |

Developing proper nutritional habits is a process; be patient with yourself. Just remember there are consequences to the way we eat. The nutrition we have today is either the "health" or "disease" we will have tomorrow.

I want you to live a long, healthy and wonderful life, so keep trying. Don't be discouraged if you occasionally slip and make bad food choices. Get back on course by making the right food choices and focus on the positive.

126

## THOUGHTS ON HEALTH AND FITNESS

* Fill your mind with positive thoughts.

* I'm going to succeed in everything I do.

* I am bigger than anything that can happen to me.

* I can do all things through Christ who strengthens me.

* If you are going to succeed, you have to feel good about yourself.

* Feed the positive and starve the negative.

* Through repetition, any action can become a habit.

* If you have faith, nothing will be impossible to you.

&ast;     &ast;     &ast;

# FAD DIETS AND DEVICES

**11**

Fad diets don't work. They don't establish long - term eating and exercise habits that lead to permanent fat loss. Following is a list of various types of fad diets and devices:

* **High protein diets** restrict carbohydrates and induces water loss, not fat loss.

* **Fasting** causes water and muscle to be lost very quickly, but not fat.

* **Diet pills** are ineffective for long - term fat loss.

* **Diets (420 - 800 calories per day)** can be dangerous and may impede fat loss.

* **Liposuction** is neither a cure for being overweight nor a substitute for healthy eating and exercise.

* **Muscle stimulators** can help rehabilitate injured muscles, but do not burn calories for fat loss.

* **Bodywraps (sauna suits, plastic wraps, and rubber jumpsuits)** lead to dehydration and a temporary water loss, but not fat loss.

## HOW TO CHANGE UNHEALTHY EATING HABITS

Changing "bad" or unhealthy eating habits is simple. The trick is to make mental associations between unhealthy habits and negative results. For example, there is an old saying that you will know a tree by its fruit. If you plant the seeds of a high-fat diet, you will produce the fruit of a high-fat body. On the other hand, if you plant the seeds of a low-fat, highly nutritious diet, you will produce the fruit of a low-fat and well-toned body. Associate negative habits with negative results and get serious about making right food choices. Eat lean and be lean. Eat healthy and be healthy. You Can Do It!

To develop healthy eating habits, it is important to never skip meals. Your body is in a dynamic state of change. You are burning calories all day long. As you burn calories, you need to replace them to keep your system functioning properly at a high energy level. Food is the gas that fuels your body. You should eat three meals and one or two snacks daily.

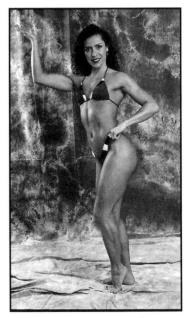

# JUNK FOOD

Remove junk food and other unhealthy foods from your kitchen. Replace them with healthy choices before you start your nutrition program. This will make the process easier. Limit your junk food intake by satisfying your "sweet tooth" with fresh fruit.

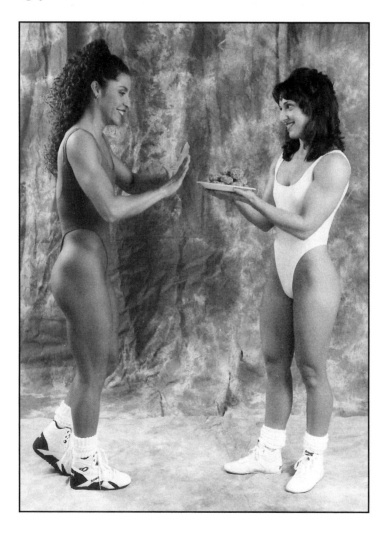

Don't be discouraged by an occasional set back. Just remember that success rarely comes in a straight line.

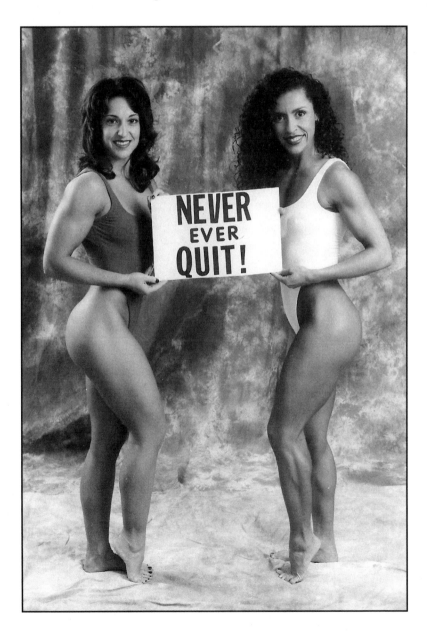

# THOUGHTS ON HEALTH FITNESS

* No one can stop you but yourself.

* Through repetition you can change any habit.

* Your greatest power is the power to choose.

* I can do everything well, including losing weight.

* Before going to sleep, fill your mind with inspiring and encouraging thoughts.

* A mind filled with sick thoughts will produce a sick body.

* Negative thoughts are thieves. They steal your health and rob you of peace of mind.

* Every evil feeling toward another is a little disease producer.

* Think and say only that which you wish to come true.

*     *     *

# 12

# CHECKING ACCOUNT FAT LOSS SYSTEM

The Checking Account Fat Loss System will guide you from where you are to where you want to be in the quickest, easiest, and safest way possible. This system uses a daily nutrition journal as well as a scale to help you determine your daily total calories, choose the right foods, and plan weekly fat loss. The Checking Account Fat Loss System will not only help you reach your goal body weight, but will also help you create healthier eating habits.

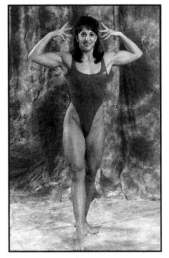

**INCH BY INCH FAT LOSS IS A CINCH**

135

# EXAMPLE:

## CHECKING ACCOUNT FAT LOSS SYSTEM

* **Step One**
  Determine your goal bodyweight
  Goal bodyweight - 140

* **Step Two**
  Determine how much you need to eat to reach your goal. Multiply your desired weight by eleven. This is the number of calories you should eat each day. Example:

  Goal bodyweight 140 Multiplied by 11 = 1540 (Daily caloric intake.) Having fewer calories can slow your metabolism and impede fat loss. Having too many calories will increase your bodyweight.

* **Step Three**
  Using the checking account system, set up a daily nutrition journal. (see pages 145-146).

  From the nutritional success formula (page 150), choose foods from the food guide calorie chart. (See pages 155-166) Record nutrition each day until you reach your goal. Write down everything you eat. This will help you identify problem areas. Gradually replace your problem foods with healthier choices.

* **Step Four**
  Set up a weekly chart of fat loss (see page 137-138). I recommend losing one pound of fat per week.

# EXAMPLE:

## WEEKLY FAT LOSS CHART

✳ Determine your weekly fat loss goals. Example:

| | |
|---|---|
| **Actual Bodyweight** | 160 |
| **Goal Bodyweight** | 140 |
| **Difference** | 20 |

✳ The difference is how many weeks it will take you to reach your goal bodyweight, if you lose one pound of fat per week.

✳ I recommend losing one pound of fat per week to guarantee long term success with the fat loss and lifestyle changes that will occur.

✳ Set weekly fat loss goals on your Weekly Fat Loss Chart.

✳ Start with present weight and subtract one pound per week until you reach your goal bodyweight on the chart.

✳ Each week fill in your actual weight next to your weekly bodyweight goal.

✳   ✳   ✳

# EXAMPLE:
## WEEKLY FAT LOSS CHART

| DATE | WEEKLY GOAL WEIGHT | ACTUAL BODYWEIGHT |
|---|---|---|
| May  6 | 0 | 160 |
| 13 | 159 | 158 |
| 20 | 158 | 157 |
| 27 | 157 | 155 |
| June  3 | 156 | 154 |
| 10 | 155 | 152 |
| 17 | 154 | 151 |
| 24 | 153 | 150 |
| July  1 | 152 | 149 |
| 8 | 151 | 147 |
| 15 | 150 | 146 |
| 22 | 149 | 145 |
| 29 | 148 | 144 |
| August  5 | 147 | 143 |
| 12 | 146 | 142 |
| 19 | 145 | 141 |
| 26 | 144 | 140 |
| September  2 | 143 | 139 |
| 9 | 142 | 138 |
| 16 | 141 | 137 |
| 23  GOAL ACHIEVED | 140 | 136 |

**REMEMBER: EACH WEEK FILL IN YOUR ACTUAL BODY-WEIGHT NEXT TO YOUR WEEKLY BODYWEIGHT GOAL**

# YOU CAN CHANGE ANYTHING

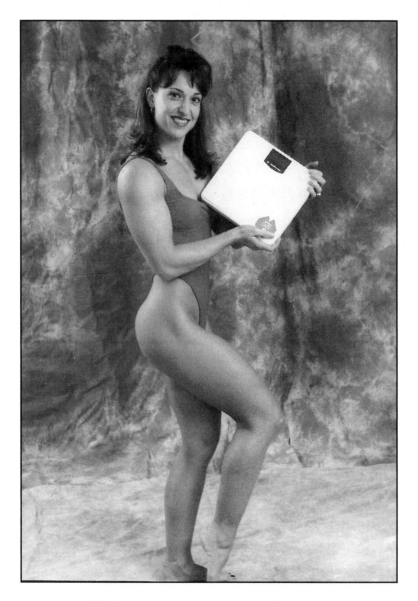

**Make the scale your friend.
Control it; don't let it control you.**

The scale is only a guide to help you reach your goal bodyweight. The true measure of fat loss is a reduction in your skirt, pants or belt size.

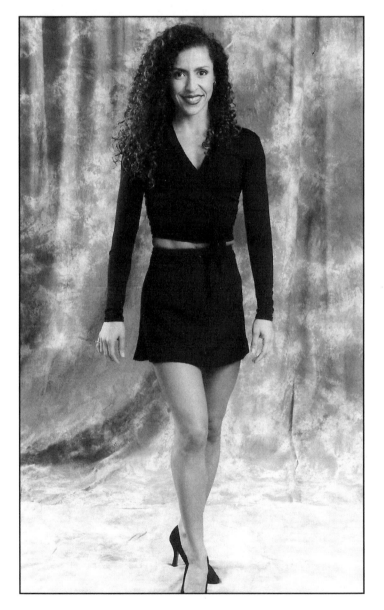

# THOUGHTS ON HEALTH FITNESS

* Stored fat on the body is the result of excessive food intake.

* Accept the idea that it is best to lose fat slowly.

* Only a scheduled fat loss and exercise program will help you reduce unwanted body fat.

* There is only one way to fail, and that is to quit.

* When you are trying, you are winning.

* Focus your efforts on one goal at a time

* Fitness is a state of mind. If you want to be fit, start thinking of yourself as fit.

* You are bigger than any problem.

* Having recognized that you have missed the mark, don't sweat it. Simply correct it and get back on course.

* Never, never, never give up.

# 13

# DAILY NUTRITION JOURNAL

The daily nutrition journal is a record of the foods you eat and their caloric content. To reach your fat loss goals, you must keep accurate records of how much food you eat each day. You start by multiplying your goal bodyweight by eleven. This will give you the number of calories you 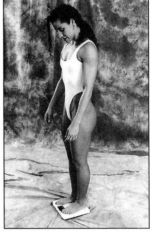 need to consume each day to reach your goal.

As you eat a meal or snack, record the foods and beverages in your journal and subtract the number of calories contained in each item from your daily total calories. Repeat this process with each meal and when you get to zero, stop eating. If you don't, any calories consumed above your daily total caloric goal will result in a weight gain.

The key to staying within your daily caloric goal is to plan your meals in advance and choose foods wisely. Don't use all of your calories up in one or two meals. The first meal is especially crucial. When you start out on the right foods, it is hard to get off track for the rest of the day. The reverse is also true.

I guarantee that you will achieve your weekly fat loss goals if you don't exceed your daily caloric intake. Remember, whenever you exceed your daily caloric intake goals, you will gain weight.

✱     ✱     ✱

## FOOD RECORDING HELPS YOU...

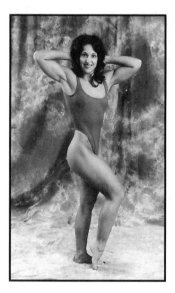

* Focus and learn about your eating style.

* Feel good about the food you eat.

* Plan your meals in advance.

* Develop a healthy food habit that will become a part of you.

* Develop your daily blue print to a successful nutrition plan.

✱     ✱     ✱

# EXAMPLE:

# DAILY NUTRITION JOURNAL

**Date:** March 4, 2000

Goal Bodyweight 140 Multiplied by 11 = 1540 (daily total calories)

## BREAKFAST

| Food | Calories |
|------|----------|
| smoked turkey breast - 4 oz | 200 |
| toasted wheat bread - 2 slices | 112 |
| banana small - 1 | 86 |
| **Remaining Calories =** | 1142 |

## SNACK

| Food | Calories |
|------|----------|
| cottage cheese - 2 oz. | 82 |
| peaches medium - 2 | 76 |
| carrots raw - 2 | 84 |
| **Remaining Calories =** | 900 |

## LUNCH

| Food | Calories |
|------|----------|
| chicken breast - 1 | 120 |
| brown rice cooked - half cup | 89 |
| broccoli cooked - 2 cups | 80 |
| **Remaining Calories =** | 611 |

## SNACK

| Food | Calories |
|------|----------|
| frozen yogurt non fat 4 oz. | 114 |
| orange medium - 2 | 128 |
| **Remaining Calories =** | 369 |

**DINNER**

| Food | Calories |
|---|---|
| Catfish - 4 oz. | 120 |
| baked potato - 1 | 76 |
| mixed vegetables - 3 cups | 100 |
| cantaloupe - half | 60 |
| **TOTAL CALORIES =** | **1527** |
| **DAILY GOAL** | **1540** |

★　　　★　　　★

# REMEMBER

★ Subtract calories for your daily total as you eat.

★ Stop eating once you get to zero balance each day or you will increase your daily total calories and this will increase your bodyweight. I guarantee you will achieve your weekly fat loss goals if you don't exceed your daily total caloric intake.

★ Focus on one day at a time.

★ Your first meal will set the pace for all your meals.

★　　　★　　　★

# CAUTION

Don't try to lose more than one pound of fat a week. Many have tried this and failed in the long run. Only an organized fat loss program will produce the long-term results you want.

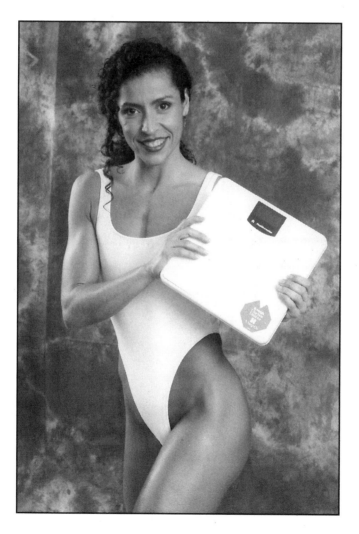

# 14

# NUTRITIONAL SUCCESS FORMULA

The nutritional success formula is a well-balanced nutritional plan that will provide your body with all the vitamins, minerals, proteins, fats and carbohydrates you need daily. Using your food guide calorie chart:

* Choose three lean meats that are four ounces per serving daily.

* Choose six cups of vegetables daily.

* Choose six pieces of fruit daily.

* Choose two low fat milk products that are six ounces each daily.

* Choose your remaining calories from grains and cereals to balance your daily caloric intake.

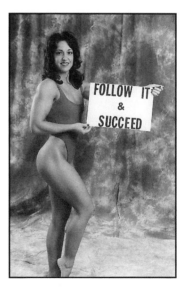

Follow this nutritional success formula daily and you will soon have the trim, healthy body you've always wanted.

# USING THE NUTRITIONAL SUCCESS FORMULA

You cannot change your eating habits in one day. Gradually you will be able to take in daily all the foods on the nutritional success formula. Concentrate on one food category each week.

**Week One**
> Choose three lean meats daily (four ounces per serving).

**Week Two**
> Choose six cups of vegetables daily.

**Week Three**
> Choose six pieces of fruit daily.

**Week Four**
> Choose two low - fat milk products daily (six ounces each).

**Week Five**
> Choose your remaining calories from grains and cereals to balance your daily caloric intake. When the fifth week is completed, start over.

\*     \*     \*

Once you can follow the nutritional success formula on a daily basis, it will become a habit and be a part of your lifestyle. This is the goal.

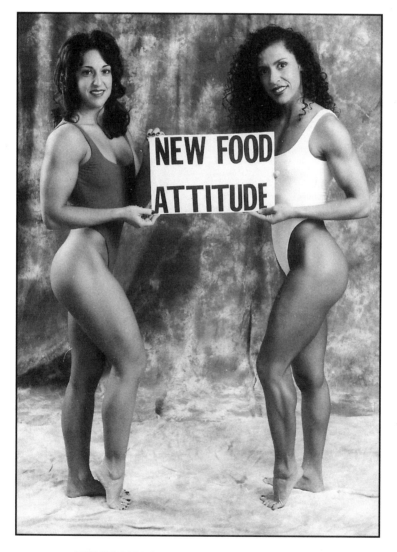

# ENJOY THE PROCESS !

# REWARDS

Select a reward for your successful completion of your fat loss goal each month.

## YOUR REWARDS EXAMPLE:

1. Movie
2. Candle light bubble bath
3. Massage
4. Manicure
5. Flowers

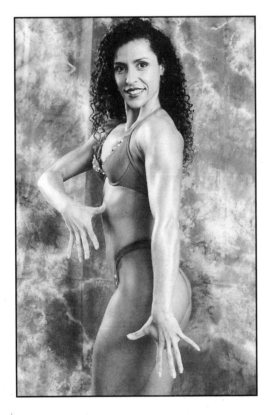

## DON'T REWARD YOURSELF WITH FOOD

# ADJUSTMENTS

Weekly adjustments will help you get back on track if you don't achieve your weekly fat loss goals. What adjustments are you going to make in your nutrition program, if you don't achieve your weekly fat loss goals? Write down your adjustment on a separate sheet of paper.

## YOUR ADJUSTMENTS EXAMPLE:

1. Get the "I can do it" attitude.
2. Avoid the situation that made you slip up.
3. Stay focused on your daily goal.
4. Remove anything that is a repeated obstacle; i.e.,...
5. Plan your daily schedule in advance.

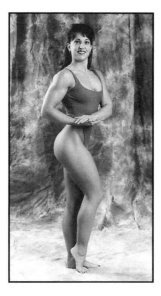

## KEEP WORKING IT!

# REMEMBER

Your goal should be to change your eating habits for a lifetime. If you go back to your old eating habits, you will regain your old weight back.

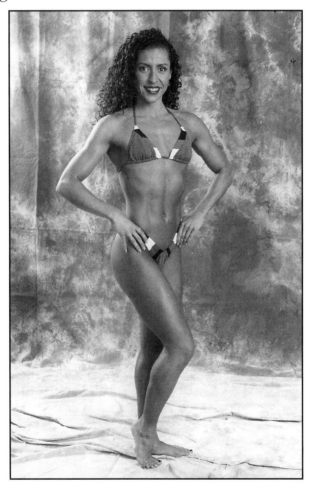

## DIETING IS TEMPORARY
## LIFESTYLE CHANGES ARE PERMANENT.

# FOOD GUIDE CALORIE CHARTS

**15**

★ Vegetable Group

★ Fruit Group

★ Grain and Cereal Group

★ Meat, Poultry & Fish Group

★ Dairy Group

★ Miscellaneous Foods

# ABBREVIATION KEY

| | | |
|---|---|---|
| C. | = | Cup/Cups |
| Oz. | = | Ounce/Ounces |
| Pc. | = | Piece |
| Pcs. | = | Pieces |
| Tbl. | = | Tablespoon/Tablespoons |
| Tsp. | = | Teaspoon/Teaspoons |

# FOOD GUIDE CALORIE CHARTS

## VEGETABLE GROUP

| Food | Qty. | Calories | Protein | Carbs. | Fat |
|---|---|---|---|---|---|
| Alfalfa sprouts, raw | 1 C. | 4 | 5.00 | 0.00 | 0.60 |
| Asparagus spears, cooked | 4 | 20 | 2.20 | 3.60 | 0.20 |
| Asparagus spears, raw | 1 C. | 35 | 3.40 | 6.80 | 0.30 |
| Bamboo shoots | 1 C. | 44 | 2.80 | 9.90 | 0.20 |
| Beets, cooked | 1 C. | 54 | 1.90 | 12.20 | 0.20 |
| Broccoli, cooked | 1 C. | 40 | 4.80 | 7.00 | 0.50 |
| Brussels sprouts, cooked | 1 C. | 56 | 6.50 | 9.90 | 0.10 |
| Cabbage, cooked | 1 C. | 29 | 1.60 | 6.20 | 0.30 |
| Cabbage, raw | 1 C. | 17 | 0.90 | 3.80 | 0.10 |
| Cabbage, steamed | 1 C. | 29 | 1.60 | 6.00 | 0.30 |
| Carrot juice | 1/2 C. | 48 | 1.24 | 11.10 | 0.00 |
| Carrots, cooked | 1 C. | 48 | 1.40 | 11.00 | 0.30 |
| Carrots, raw | 1 | 42 | 1.00 | 10.00 | 0.20 |
| Cauliflower, cooked | 1 C. | 28 | 2.90 | 5.10 | 0.30 |
| Cauliflower, raw | 1 C. | 27 | 2.70 | 5.20 | 0.20 |
| Celery, cooked | 1 C. | 21 | 1.20 | 4.70 | 0.20 |
| Celery, raw | 1 C. | 20 | 1.10 | 14.70 | 0.10 |
| Chard, Swiss, cooked | 1 C. | 26 | 2.60 | 4.80 | 0.30 |
| Chard, raw | 1 C. | 25 | 2.40 | 4.60 | 0.30 |
| Collards, cooked | 1 C. | 42 | 3.90 | 7.10 | 0.90 |
| Collards, raw | 1 C. | 40 | 3.60 | 7.20 | 0.70 |
| Corn | 1/2 C. | 66 | 1.53 | 13.33 | 0.60 |
| Corn on the cob | 1 | 70 | 1.20 | 15.80 | 0.30 |
| Cucumber raw | 1 C. | 16 | 0.90 | 3.60 | 0.10 |
| Dandelion greens, cooked | 1 C. | 35 | 2.10 | 6.70 | 0.60 |
| Egg plant, baked | 1 C. | 38 | 2.00 | 8.20 | 0.40 |
| Kale, cooked | 1 C. | 43 | 5.00 | 6.70 | 0.80 |
| Kale, raw | 1 C. | 38 | 4.20 | 6.00 | 0.80 |
| Lettuce, chopped | 2 C. | 20 | 1.40 | 4.00 | 0.20 |
| Minestrone soup | 1/2 C. | 53 | 2.50 | 7.00 | 1.70 |
| Mushrooms | 1 C. | 20 | 2.00 | 3.00 | 3.70 |

| Food | Qty. | Calories | Protein | Carbs. | Fat |
|------|------|----------|---------|--------|-----|
| Mushrooms, medium, sauteed | 2 | 39 | 0.85 | 1.40 | 3.70 |
| Mustard greens, cooked | 1 C. | 29 | 3.10 | 5.00 | 0.40 |
| Mustard greens, raw | 3.5 oz. | 31 | 3.00 | 5.60 | 0.50 |
| Okra, cooked | 1 C. | 46 | 3.20 | 9.60 | 0.50 |
| Okra, raw | 1 C. | 36 | 2.40 | 7.60 | 0.30 |
| Onions, chopped, raw | 1/2 C. | 32 | 1.30 | 7.40 | 0.10 |
| Onions, cooked | 1 C. | 61 | 2.50 | 13.70 | 0.20 |
| Parsnips, cooked | 6 Oz. | 76 | 1.73 | 17.33 | 0.60 |
| Parsnip, raw | 1/2 | 76 | 1.70 | 17.50 | 0.50 |
| Peas, cooked | 1/2 C. | 57 | 4.30 | 9.70 | 0.30 |
| Potato, plain, baked with skin | 1/2 | 72 | 2.00 | 16.50 | 0.10 |
| Potato, plain, boiled with skin | 1 | 76 | 2.10 | 17.10 | 0.10 |
| Potatoes, french fried | 5 Pcs. | 69 | 1.05 | 9.00 | 3.30 |
| Potatoes, mashed with milk | 1/2 C. | 69 | 2.20 | 13.60 | 1.50 |
| Pumpkin, canned | 1/2 C. | 41 | 1.25 | 9.70 | 0.30 |
| Red cabbage, raw | 1 C. | 22 | 1.40 | 4.80 | 0.10 |
| Rutabaga, cooked | 1 C. | 60 | 1.50 | 13.90 | 0.20 |
| Rutabaga, raw | 1 C. | 64 | 1.50 | 15.40 | 0.10 |
| Sauerkraut | 1 C. | 42 | 2.40 | 9.40 | 0.50 |
| Soup, split pea | 1/2 C. | 74 | 4.40 | 10.50 | 1.65 |
| Spinach, cooked | 1 C. | 41 | 5.40 | 6.50 | 0.50 |
| Spinach, raw | 1 C. | 14 | 1.80 | 2.40 | 0.20 |
| Squash, summer, cooked | 1 C. | 25 | 1.60 | 5.60 | 0.20 |
| Squash, winter, baked | 1/2 C. | 65 | 1.85 | 15.80 | 0.40 |
| String beans | 1 C. | 22 | 1.40 | 3.60 | 0.20 |
| Sweet potato, baked | 1/2 | 80 | 1.20 | 18.50 | 0.30 |
| Tomato, large | 1/2 | 17 | 0.80 | 4.00 | 0.20 |
| Tomato juice | 1 C. | 46 | 2.20 | 10.40 | 0.20 |
| Tomato sauce | 2 oz. | 54 | 2.25 | 12.25 | 0.25 |
| Turnips, cooked | 1 C. | 36 | 1.20 | 7.60 | 0.30 |
| V-8 juice | 1 C. | 41 | 2.00 | 9.00 | 0.20 |
| Watercress, raw | 1 C. | 7 | 0.80 | 1.10 | 0.10 |

★ ★ ★

# FRUIT GROUP

| Food | Qty. | Calories | Protein | Carbs. | Fat |
|------|------|----------|---------|--------|-----|
| Apple, medium | 1/2 | 48 | 0.15 | 12.00 | 0.50 |
| Apple juice | 1/2 C. | 59 | 0.10 | 14.75 | 0.00 |
| Apple sauce | 1/2 C. | 50 | 0.25 | 11.50 | 0.25 |
| Apricots, average, raw | 3 | 55 | 1.10 | 13.70 | 0.20 |
| Apricot nectar | 1/2 C. | 71 | 0.40 | 18.30 | 0.30 |
| Avocado | 1 | 34 | 0.40 | 1.20 | 3.20 |
| Banana, small | 1/2 | 43 | 0.53 | 11.10 | 0.10 |
| Blackberries, raw | 1/2 C. | 42 | 0.85 | 9.30 | 0.65 |
| Blueberries, raw | 1/2 C. | 45 | 0.50 | 11.00 | 0.40 |
| Cantaloupe | 1/2 | 60 | 1.40 | 15.00 | 0.20 |
| Cherries, sweet, raw | 1/2 C. | 41 | 0.75 | 10.20 | 0.20 |
| Dates, pitted | 2 | 55 | 0.44 | 14.58 | 0.10 |
| Fig, dried | 1 | 55 | 0.86 | 13.82 | 0.26 |
| Fig, fresh | 1 | 40 | 0.60 | 10.15 | 0.12 |
| Fruit juice | 1/2 C. | 61 | 0.85 | 14.50 | 0.10 |
| Fruit salad | 1/2 C. | 45 | 1.00 | 10.15 | 0.12 |
| Grape juice | 1/2 C. | 83 | 0.25 | 21.00 | 0.00 |
| Grapefruit juice | 1/2 C. | 49 | 0.60 | 11.50 | 0.10 |
| Grapefruit, medium | 1/2 | 41 | 0.50 | 11.00 | 0.10 |
| Grapes | 1/2 C. | 53 | 1.00 | 12.00 | 0.00 |
| Honeydew melon slice, raw | 2 in. | 49 | 1.20 | 11.50 | 0.50 |
| Lemon juice | 9 Tbl. | 36 | 0.90 | 10.80 | 0.00 |
| Mango fruit, chopped | 1/2 | 76 | 0.80 | 19.40 | 0.45 |
| Nectarine, medium | 1/2 | 44 | 0.40 | 11.60 | 0.00 |
| Orange, medium | 1 | 64 | 1.30 | 16.00 | 0.30 |
| Orange juice | 1/2 C. | 61 | 1.00 | 14.50 | 0.10 |
| Papaya fruit, medium | 1/2 | 58 | 0.90 | 15.00 | 0.15 |
| Peach, medium | 1 | 38 | 0.60 | 9.70 | 0.10 |
| Pear, large | 1/2 | 61 | 0.70 | 15.30 | 0.40 |
| Pineapple | 1/2 C. | 90 | 0.60 | 22.00 | 0.20 |
| Pineapple juice | 1/2 C. | 69 | 0.50 | 16.60 | 0.15 |
| Plums, medium | 2 | 66 | 0.50 | 17.80 | 0.00 |
| Prunes, dry | 2 | 50 | 0.50 | 13.30 | 0.10 |
| Raisins | 1 C. | 48 | 0.41 | 12.80 | 0.03 |
| Raspberries, black raw | 1/2 C. | 49 | 1.00 | 10.50 | 0.95 |

| Food | Qty. | Calories | Protein | Carbs. | Fat |
|------|------|----------|---------|--------|-----|
| Raspberries, red, raw | 1 C. | 70 | 1.50 | 16.70 | 0.60 |
| Strawberries | 1 C. | 39 | 0.70 | 10.00 | 0.20 |
| Tangerine, medium | 1 | 39 | 0.70 | 10.00 | 0.20 |
| Watermelon | 1 C. | 45 | 0.50 | 10.00 | 0.20 |

★    ★    ★

# GRAIN AND CEREAL GROUP

| Food | Qty. | Calories | Protein | Carbs. | Fat |
|------|------|----------|---------|--------|-----|
| Beans, baked | 1/3 C. | 75 | 4.80 | 13.50 | 0.30 |
| Biscuit | 1/2 | 53 | 1.05 | 6.40 | 2.40 |
| Bran flakes, 40% fortified | 1/2 C. | 53 | 1.80 | 14.10 | 0.30 |
| Bread, cracked wheat | 1 Slice | 60 | 2.00 | 12.00 | 0.60 |
| Bread, pumpernickel | 1 Slice | 79 | 2.90 | 17.00 | 0.40 |
| Bread, raisin | 1 Slice | 60 | 1.50 | 12.64 | 0.00 |
| Bread, rye | 1 Slice | 56 | 2.10 | 12.00 | 1.00 |
| Bread, white enriched | 1 Slice | 62 | 2.00 | 11.60 | 0.20 |
| Bread, whole wheat | 1 Slice | 56 | 2.40 | 11.00 | 0.79 |
| Bread, whole wheat, toast | 1 Slice | 60 | 2.00 | 12.00 | 0.50 |
| Bun, burger or hot-dog | 1/2 | 60 | 1.65 | 10.60 | 1.10 |
| Cereal, cooked | 1/2 C. | 67 | 2.25 | 14.00 | 0.20 |
| Cereal, dry | 1/2 C. | 53 | 1.75 | 14.00 | 0.25 |
| Corn bread | 1 Pc. | 93 | 3.30 | 13.10 | 3.20 |
| Corn flakes, dry cereal | 1/2 C. | 49 | 1.00 | 10.50 | 0.05 |
| Corn grits, hominy, cooked | 1/2 C. | 63 | 1.45 | 13.50 | 0.12 |
| Corn meal, enriched, cooked | 1/2 C. | 60 | 1.20 | 12.58 | 0.25 |
| Crackers, graham plain | 1 | 55 | 1.10 | 10.40 | 1.30 |
| Crackers, soda | 5 | 63 | 1.30 | 10.00 | 1.85 |
| Cream of wheat | 1/2 C. | 67 | 2.25 | 14.00 | 0.12 |
| Granola | 1/2 C. | 78 | 1.80 | 11.40 | 3.00 |
| Macaroni, enriched, cooked | 1/2 C. | 75 | 2.40 | 16.10 | 0.50 |
| Muffin, bran | 1 | 104 | 3.00 | 17.00 | 4.00 |
| Muffin, English, toasted | 1/2 | 59 | 1.65 | 8.45 | 2.00 |
| Muffin, plain, enriched | 1/2 | 59 | 1.55 | 8.45 | 2.00 |
| Muffin, whole wheat | 1/2 | 52 | 2.00 | 10.45 | 0.55 |
| Noodles, egg, enriched | 1/2 C. | 100 | 3.30 | 18.65 | 1.20 |
| Oat flakes, fortified | 1/2 C. | 74 | 3.34 | 13.40 | 1.05 |
| Oatmeal | 1/2 C. | 66 | 2.40 | 11.51 | 1.40 |

| Food | Qty. | Calories | Protein | Carbs. | Fat |
|---|---|---|---|---|---|
| Pancake, buckwheat | 1 | 54 | 1.80 | 6.40 | 2.50 |
| Pancake, plain, enriched | 1 | 62 | 2.00 | 9.00 | 2.00 |
| Pancake, whole wheat | 1 | 74 | 3.40 | 8.80 | 3.20 |
| Pasta, whole wheat, dry | 1 Oz. | 100 | 5.00 | 19.50 | 0.03 |
| Pita, whole wheat average | 1/2 | 70 | 3.00 | 12.00 | 1.00 |
| Popcorn, plain | 1 C. | 54 | 1.80 | 10.70 | 0.70 |
| Rice, brown | 1/2 C. | 89 | 2.00 | 19.00 | 0.60 |
| Rice, brown, cooked | 1/2 C. | 89 | 1.90 | 19.10 | 0.60 |
| Rice, cooked | 1/2 C. | 9 | 1.50 | 18.00 | 0.10 |
| Rice, puffed, fortified | 1 C. | 60 | 0.90 | 13.40 | 0.10 |
| Roll, dinner | 1 | 89 | 2.50 | 16.00 | 1.70 |
| Roll, French | 1 | 113 | 3.00 | 20.00 | 2.00 |
| Roll, whole wheat | 1/2 | 78 | 2.50 | 15.00 | 0.80 |
| Roll, whole wheat | 1 | 90 | 3.50 | 18.30 | 0.30 |
| Crackers, Ryekrisp | 3 | 63 | 2.40 | 14.40 | 0.22 |
| Shredded wheat, biscuit | 1 | 89 | 2.50 | 20.00 | 0.50 |
| Spaghetti, cooked | 1/2 C. | 75 | 2.50 | 16.00 | 0.25 |
| Tortilla, yellow corn | 1 | 63 | 1.50 | 13.50 | 0.60 |
| Wheat, flakes, fortified | 1/2 C. | 53 | 1.55 | 12.10 | 0.36 |
| Wheat, puffed, fortified | 1 C. | 54 | 2.30 | 11.80 | 0.70 |
| Yams, cooked in skin | 3 Oz. | 90 | 2.06 | 20.66 | 0.17 |

★       ★       ★

# MEAT, POULTRY AND FISH GROUP

| Food | Qty. | Calories | Protein | Carbs. | Fat |
|------|------|----------|---------|--------|-----|
| Abalone | 4 Oz. | 111 | 21.20 | 3.85 | 0.58 |
| Bass | 4 Oz. | 118 | 21.43 | 0.00 | 2.39 |
| Beef, flank steak | 3 Oz | 122 | 18.38 | 0.00 | 4.86 |
| Beef, ground round | 2 Oz. | 102 | 11.75 | 0.00 | 5.50 |
| Beef, lean cut | 2 Oz. | 125 | 16.00 | 0.00 | 7.00 |
| Beef, lean ground | 2 Oz. | 102 | 12.00 | 0.00 | 5.50 |
| Beef, lean steak | 2 Oz. | 108 | 11.06 | 0.00 | 6.74 |
| Canadian bacon | 2 Oz. | 123 | 11.50 | 0.20 | 8.00 |
| Catfish | 4 Oz | 117 | 19.95 | 0.00 | 3.52 |
| Chicken breast, baked | 4 Oz. | 99 | 18.50 | 0.00 | 4.50 |
| Clams, large | 6 | 99 | 18.50 | 0.00 | 4.50 |
| Cod | 5 Oz. | 123 | 21.00 | 1.95 | 2.85 |
| Cold cuts | 2 Oz. | 111 | 24.94 | 0.00 | 1.03 |
| Crab meat | 3 Oz. | 71 | 15.60 | 0.00 | 0.51 |
| Flounder | 5 Oz. | 112 | 31.67 | 0.00 | 1.72 |
| Frog legs, large | 6 | 110 | 24.60 | 0.00 | 0.45 |
| Haddock | 5 Oz. | 112 | 25.94 | 0.00 | 0.93 |
| Halibut | 4 Oz. | 114 | 23.70 | 0.00 | 1.25 |
| Ham, sliced | 2 Oz. | 125 | 16.00 | 0.00 | 7.00 |
| Lamb | 2 Oz. | 125 | 16.00 | 0.00 | 7.00 |
| Liver | 8 Oz. | 117 | 10.00 | 2.65 | 8.65 |
| Lobster | 4 Oz. | 103 | 19.18 | 0.58 | 2.15 |
| Oysters, fresh | 6 Oz. | 112 | 14.28 | 5.78 | 3.08 |
| Perch, ocean | 4 Oz. | 108 | 21.55 | 0.00 | 2.83 |
| Perch, yellow | 4 Oz. | 103 | 22.13 | 0.00 | 1.03 |
| Pollock, filet | 4 Oz. | 108 | 23.13 | 0.00 | 1.03 |
| Red snapper | 4 Oz. | 106 | 22.50 | 0.00 | 1.38 |
| Salmon, fresh | 2 Oz. | 123 | 12.75 | 0.00 | 7.60 |
| Sandabs | 5 Oz. | 112 | 31.67 | 0.00 | 1.72 |
| Sardines, canned, drained | 2 Oz. | 116 | 13.60 | 0.00 | 6.20 |
| Scallops | 5 Oz. | 115 | 21.69 | 4.69 | 0.28 |
| Shrimps, canned, drained | 1 C. | 148 | 31.00 | 0.90 | 1.40 |
| Shrimps, fresh | 4 Oz. | 103 | 20.53 | 1.70 | 0.90 |
| Snails | 4 Oz. | 103 | 18.40 | 2.29 | 1.60 |

| Food | Qty. | Calories | Protein | Carbs. | Fat |
|---|---|---|---|---|---|
| Sole | 5 Oz. | 112 | 31.67 | 0.00 | 1.72 |
| Swordfish | 4 Oz. | 134 | 21.78 | 0.00 | 4.52 |
| Trout, rainbow | 2 Oz. | 111 | 12.19 | 0.00 | 6.46 |
| Tuna, water-packed | 4 Oz. | 127 | 28.00 | 0.00 | 0.80 |
| Turkey, skinned, baked | 2 Oz. | 104 | 21.00 | 0.00 | 2.25 |
| Turkey breast | 2 Oz. | 100 | 18.50 | 0.00 | 2.25 |

★ ★ ★

# DAIRY GROUP

| Food | Qty. | Calories | Protein | Carbs. | Fat |
|------|------|----------|---------|--------|-----|
| Butter | 1/2 Tbl. | 51 | 0.05 | 0.05 | 6.30 |
| Butter | 1 Tsp. | 33 | 0.10 | 0.00 | 4.00 |
| Buttermilk | 1.5 C. | 149 | 12.15 | 17.55 | 3.24 |
| Cheese, cheddar | 1 Oz | 168 | 10.50 | 0.60 | 14.10 |
| Cheese, jack | 1 Oz | 159 | 10.50 | 0.30 | 12.90 |
| Cheese, melted | 1 Oz. | 112 | 7.00 | 0.40 | 9.00 |
| Cheese, monterey | 1 Oz. | 159 | 10.41 | 0.29 | 12.87 |
| Cheese, mozzarella | 1 Oz. | 178 | 11.00 | 1.20 | 12.00 |
| Cheese, Swiss | 1 Oz. | 107 | 8.06 | 0.96 | 7.78 |
| Cottage cheese | 4 Oz. | 163 | 19.50 | 4.20 | 7.13 |
| Egg, boiled | 1 | 82 | 6.50 | 0.50 | 6.00 |
| Egg, omlet | 1 | 111 | 7.20 | 1.50 | 7.08 |
| Egg, poached | 1 | 8 | 6.50 | 0.50 | 6.00 |
| Egg, scrambled | 1 | 82 | 6.50 | 0.05 | 6.00 |
| Egg whites | 5 | 85 | 18.00 | 1.50 | 0.00 |
| Margarine, regular | 1/2 Tbl. | 51 | 0.05 | 0.05 | 5.75 |
| Margarine, whipped | 1/2 Tbl. | 34 | 0.05 | 0.00 | 3.80 |
| Milk, goat, whole | 6 Oz. | 126 | 6.52 | 8.18 | 4.88 |
| Milk, low-fat | 1 C. | 121 | 8.12 | 11.70 | 4.68 |
| Milk, non-fat | 1 C. | 129 | 12.00 | 18.00 | 0.68 |
| Milk, whole | 6 Oz. | 119 | 6.38 | 9.00 | 6.60 |
| Sherbet | 1/2 C. | 135 | 1.08 | 29.35 | 1.91 |
| Sour cream | 1 Tbl. | 53 | 1.10 | 0.10 | 5.30 |
| Yogurt, frozen, non-fat | 4 Oz. | 114 | 4.00 | 24.00 | 0.28 |
| Yogurt, low-fat, plain | 8 Oz. | 144 | 11.90 | 16.00 | 3.52 |
| Yogurt, skim, plain | 8 Oz. | 127 | 13.00 | 17.40 | 0.41 |
| Yogurt, whole milk, plain | 8 Oz. | 139 | 7.88 | 10.60 | 7.38 |

★        ★        ★

# MISCELLANEOUS

| Food | Qty. | Calories | Protein | Carbs. | Fat |
|------|------|----------|---------|--------|-----|
| Mayonnaise | 1 Tbl. | 45 | 0.20 | 0.30 | 5.00 |
| Nuts, Macadamia | 3 | 55 | 0.70 | 0.75 | 5.85 |
| Oil, safflower | 1/2 Tbl. | 63 | 0.00 | 0.00 | 7.00 |
| Salad dressing, bleu cheese | 1/2 Tbl. | 38 | 0.35 | 0.55 | 3.90 |
| Salad dressing, French | 1/2 Tbl. | 33 | 0.50 | 1.40 | 3.10 |
| Salad dressing, Italian | 1/2 Tbl. | 42 | 0.00 | 0.50 | 9.00 |
| Salad dressing, Russian | 1/2 Tbl. | 37 | 0.10 | 0.80 | 3.80 |
| Salad dressing, thousand island | 1/2 Tbl. | 40 | 0.05 | 1.25 | 4.00 |
| Salad dressing, thousand island, low calorie | 2 Tbl. | 54 | 0.20 | 4.60 | 4.20 |
| Soup, cream of celery | 1/2 C. | 43 | 1.00 | 4.50 | 2.50 |
| Soup, cream of chicken | 1/2 C. | 47 | 1.50 | 4.00 | 3.00 |

★　　　★　　　★

# CHARTS

## 16

★    Weekly Exercise Record

★    Weekly Fat Loss Chart

★    Daily Nutrition Journal

# SAMPLE

## WEEKLY EXERCISE RECORD

### Week of _____

| | Body-shaping | Weights | Aerobics exercise | Time | Notes |
|------|------|------|------|------|------|
| MON | | | | | |
| TUES | | | | | |
| WED | | | | | |
| THUR | | | | | |
| FRI | | | | | |
| SAT | | | | | |
| SUN | | | | | |

## RECORD FOR SUCCESS

★     ★     ★

# WEEKLY FAT LOSS CHART

* Determine your weekly fat loss goals.

   **Actual bodyweight**  _____

   **Goal bodyweight**  _____

   **Difference**  _____

* The difference is how many weeks it will take you to reach your goal bodyweight if you lose one pound of fat per week.

* I recommend losing one pound of fat per week to guarantee long-term success with the fat loss and lifestyle changes that occur.

* Set weekly fat loss goals on your Weekly Fat Loss Chart.

* Start with your present weight and subtract one pound each week until you reach your goal bodyweight on the chart.

* Each week fill in your actual weight next to your weekly bodyweight goal.

★      ★      ★

# SAMPLE:
# WEEKLY FAT LOSS CHART

| DATE | WEEKLY GOAL WEIGHT | ACTUAL BODYWEIGHT |
|------|--------------------|--------------------|
|      |                    |                    |
|      |                    |                    |
|      |                    |                    |
|      |                    |                    |
|      |                    |                    |
|      |                    |                    |
|      |                    |                    |
|      |                    |                    |
|      |                    |                    |
|      |                    |                    |
|      |                    |                    |
|      |                    |                    |
|      |                    |                    |
|      |                    |                    |
|      |                    |                    |
|      |                    |                    |
|      |                    |                    |
|      |                    |                    |
|      |                    |                    |
|      |                    |                    |

**REMEMBER: EACH WEEK FILL IN YOUR ACTUAL BODY-WEIGHT NEXT TO YOUR WEEKLY BODYWEIGHT GOAL**

# DAILY NUTRITION JOURNAL

**Date:** _____

Goal Bodyweight _____ Multiplied by 11 = _____
(daily total calories)

## BREAKFAST
**Food**                                    **Calories**




**Remaining Calories =**          _____

## SNACK
**Food**                                    **Calories**




**Remaining Calories =**          _____

## LUNCH
**Food**                                    **Calories**




**Remaining Calories =**          _____

**SNACK**
  Food                                    **Calories**


        **Remaining Calories =**          _____

**DINNER**
  Food                                    **Calories**




        **TOTAL CALORIES =**              _____
        **DAILY GOAL**                    _____

               ✶        ✶        ✶

## REMEMBER

✶ Subtract calories for your daily total as you eat.

✶ Stop eating once you get to zero balance each day or you will increase your daily total calories and this will increase your bodyweight. I guarantee you will achieve your weekly fat loss goals if you don't exceed your daily total caloric intake.

✶ Focus on one day at a time.

✶ Your first meal will set the pace for all your meals.

               ✶        ✶        ✶

# 17

# QUESTIONS AND ANSWERS

## FAT LOSS AND NUTRITION

**Question:** What is obesity?

**Answer:** Technically, obesity is when your bodyfat is over 30 percent.

**Question:** Are there any health problems associated with being overweight?

**Answer:** If you are overweight, your chances of developing chronic health problems increase. Problems for overfat people include: heart disease, high blood pressure, diabetes, and some forms of cancer. You should focus on maintaining your ideal bodyweight.

**Question:** I think I am genetically fat. What can I do about it?

**Answer:** You may be genetically predisposed to becoming fat, but you can change your body fat composition with good nutrition, daily walks, and bodyshaping.

**Question:** What is the best way to lose weight and keep it off?

**Answer:** The best way to do this is to gradually make changes in your lifestyle so that bodyshaping, aerobics, and good nutrition become a part of your life. Dieting is temporary. Lifestyle changes are permanent.

**Question:** Why do people sometimes lose inches, rather than pounds?

**Answer:** Lost inches represent fat loss and increased pounds represent muscle gains. By eating less and exercising more, you burn your fat storage and lose inches from your body. Muscles weigh more than fat. Therefore, you can gain muscle from your exercise program, lose body fat from your nutrition program, and still maintain your starting bodyweight.

**Question:** Why am I losing dress sizes, and not losing weight?

**Answer:** You have changed your body composition, which means you have increased muscle mass and decreased body fat while maintaining the same bodyweight. You can use the scale as a measuring point, but the final decision goes to your mirror and your reduced dress size.

**Question:** Does drinking water help you lose weight?

**Answer:** Water will not rid your body of fat. The way to lose fat is to take in fewer calories than you burn.

**Question:** How do you lose one pound of body fat?

**Answer:** A reduction of 3500 calories, either through nutrition or burned in exercise, will result in a one pound body fat loss.

**Question:** Will I reach my weight loss goals quicker if I try to lose 2 to 3 pounds per week?

**Answer:** When you lose weight quickly, 50 percent of the weight loss is lean muscle, not fat. The key is to lose one pound of fat per week, through balanced nutrition, daily aerobics, and bodyshaping. This will increase your lean muscle mass while you burn off the fat.

**Question:** Why am I gaining weight eating low-fat and fat-free foods?

**Answer:** Your daily caloric intake is too high. Multiply your goal bodyweight by eleven. This will give you your daily caloric intake. Any calories eaten above your daily calorie intake will be stored as fat.

**Question:** Can I lose weight by simply cutting the fat out of my diet?

**Answer:** Reducing fat will improve the quality of your nutrition. However, any calories consumed over your weight maintenance level will be stored as fat.

**Question:** Is a high-protein diet okay?

**Answer:** High-protein diets restrict carbohydrates and this will induce water loss, not fat loss. This condition is dangerous and leads to dehydration. Your brain needs carbohydrates to function properly. Balanced nutrition is the key to long-term success.

**Question:** What is the difference between good fat and bad fat?

**Answer:** There are saturated fats and unsaturated fats. The bad fat (saturated) is solid at room temperature. Saturated fats remain solid in your arteries as well and create a clogging effect. On the other hand, unsaturated fat is liquid at room temperature and it does not have the tendency to clog the arteries.

**Question:** How can I make low-fat foods taste better?

**Answer:** The key is your imagination. Use herbs and spices, mixed with your creativity to make foods taste better.

**Question:** At what time should I stop eating at night?

**Answer:** There is no set time to stop eating. Your last meal should be two to three hours before going to bed. You will sleep more comfortably.

**Question:** Will I need special food for this program?

**Answer:** No. Ordinary, low-fat foods from the grocery store are great.

★ ★ ★

# BODYSHAPING

**Question:** Will exercising every day help me get in shape quicker?

**Answer:** Rest days are important in any exercise program. When you rest, you get results.

**Question:** Is there any truth to the saying, "no pain, no gain?"

**Answer:** Pain is the first sign of injury. If you experience pain during exercise, stop exercising immediately.

**Question:** What will happen if I go about my program without setting a goal?

**Answer:** Goals give you something for which to aim. If you don't have a measurable goal to aim for, you will miss it every time. Consequently, you will not have confidence in your program and you will not stick with it. Goals keep you going forward.

**Question:** Do women who exercise lose their femininity?

**Answer:** To the contrary, women who exercise are more feminine. They are also more shapely, confident and sexy.

**Question:** Will exercise improve my love life?

**Answer:** Yes. A fit and healthy body is a delight to the eyes and a joy to touch.

**Question:** Is it okay to take time off from exercising?

**Answer:** When you need extra rest, you should take it. Resting should be a part of your exercise program. Don't exercise every day. Think long-term success.

**Question:** Will I get big muscles from the bodyshaping workout?

**Answer:** No. Women don't produce enough of the muscle building hormone (testosterone) to develop large muscles. The bodyshaping workout will, however, shape and tone and tighten your body.

**Question:** If I stop working out, will my muscles turn to fat?

**Answer:** No. Muscle cannot turn into fat, and fat cannot turn into muscle. When you exercise, you change the shape and tone of your body and decrease body fat. When you stop, you again change the shape and tone of your body by increasing your body fat.

**Question:** Should I exercise with lower back pain?

**Answer:** Eighty-five percent of all women will experience lower back pain at one time or another. If you do, check with your physician before exercising.

**Question:** Should I exercise when I have menstrual cramps?

**Answer:** Yes, the benefits you are receiving from exercise far outweigh the possible negative factors. Keep exercising.

**Question:** Is it safe for senior citizens to exercise?

**Answer:** Exercise is great for everyone. Exercise will give you a more youthful appearance, strength and stamina.

**Question:** What if I am so weak that even without weights, I can only do a few repetitions on the bodyshaping program?

**Answer:** No problem. Focus on doing the exercises without weights until you can do the required number of repetitions on each exercise. Then, gradually start to use weights. A little weakness, when starting out, is normal but temporary.

**Question:** How will I know if I'm getting fit?

**Answer:** You will be stronger; there will be a reduction in your resting heart rate and weight.

**Question:** Why should I keep records for bodyshaping, and aerobics, as well as a food journal?

**Answer:** You will have a map of your success. If you get off track you will know exactly what to do to get back on track. The goal of self-monitoring is to help you develop an internal awareness.

&#42;    &#42;    &#42;

## SUPPLEMENTS

**Question:** When I exercise do I need more iron?

**Answer:** You don't need to increase iron because of exercise. All women can help to protect themselves from becoming iron deficient by eating a balanced diet rich in meats, fish, and chicken, all of which have iron that is absorbed by the body easily.

**Question:** Can I increase my energy with vitamin and mineral supplements?

**Answer:** Vitamin and mineral supplements do not provide calories and they cannot be used for energy. The best sources of vitamins and minerals are in the foods you eat. Always consult your physician before taking any supplements.

**Question:** Will diet pills help me loss weight?

**Answer:** Diet pills are ineffective for long-term weight loss because they don't help you change your eating habits and lifestyle.

★     ★     ★

Dear Reader,

Please write me when *Jerry Anderson's Joy of Fitness for Women* has helped you meet your fat loss and fitness goals. Include a before and after photograph, as well as any unanswered questions you may have.

I look forward to hearing from you soon.

Apex Fitness House
4102 Orange Ave.
Suite 107-183
Long Beach, CA 90807

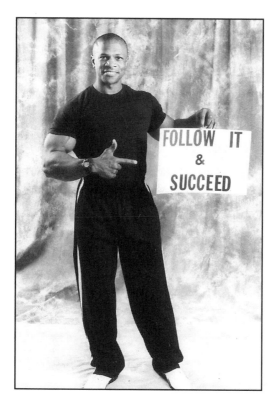

Do you know someone who will be helped by reading *Jerry Anderson's Joy of Fitness for Women*? For additional copies or to contact Jerry Anderson please write to:

Apex Fitness House
4102 Orange Ave.
Suite 107-183
Long Beach, CA 90807

*JERRY ANDERSON'S JOY OF FITNESS FOR WOMEN* is available for $24.95 plus $3.50 shipping and handling for first book. For additional books mailed to the same address there will be a $1.50 shipping and handling fee per book. (California orders please add sales tax.)

Send one to a friend...